# Diagnosis and Treatment of Global Aphasia

## CLINICAL UPDATES IN SPEECH-LANGUAGE PATHOLOGY SERIES

### Notes from an Advisory Editor

The heart of speech-language-hearing pathology is clinical practice. For the most part, clinical practitioners have had to create clinical procedures out of the stuff of their own practice or from the hints contained in general books on each of the disorders. Until now. The *Clinical Updates Series* changes that. Each book in this series emphasizes daily clinical practice. The emphasis is on how to do evaluation and treatment. Of course, the books are cookbooks. They are not grocery lists, however, nor are they esoteric analyses of cultural differences about what is edible. Readers will find discussions of specific techniques and specific guidelines for selecting and ordering materials and procedures. These books are proof that good clinicians can be good writers. They are written with the knowledge that good clinicians are like good cooks—they use what they like and need, and they adapt and change as appropriate. And they always double the mushrooms.

*Jay Rosenbek*

# Diagnosis and Treatment of Global Aphasia

**Michael Collins, Ph.D.**

*Veterans Administration Medical Center*
*Madison, Wisconsin*

*Adjunct Associate Professor*
*Department of Communicative Disorders*
*University of Wisconsin, Madison*
*Madison, Wisconsin*

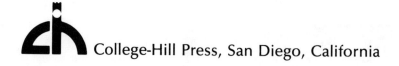
College-Hill Press, San Diego, California

College-Hill Press, Inc.
4284 41st Street
San Diego, California 92105

**Library of Congress Cataloging in Publication Data**
Main entry under title:

Collins, Michael, 1943–
   Diagnosis and treatment of global aphasia.

   Includes index.
   1. Aphasia.   2. Speech therapy.   I. Title.
   [DNLM: 1. Aphasia—diagnosis.   2. Aphasia—therapy.
   WL 340.5 C712s]
   RC425.C63   1986        616.85′52        85-30735

**ISBN 0-88744-207-2**

**Printed in the United States of America**

# CONTENTS

*For Charlie and Matt*

# Preface

The study of aphasia is the domain of a very special assembly of representatives from disparate disciplines. These representatives include speech and language pathologists, linguists, neurologists, neurolinguists, psychologists and neuropsychologists. Their territories and their responsibilities are not evenly apportioned and frequently overlap, and there seem to be few attempts to regulate the dominion of each. Instead, a rather loose academic and clinical gathering has evolved in which the well-being of aphasic patients and the accumulation of theoretical, longitudinal and clinical information to benefit our aphasic patients are paramount.

This catholic and eclectic group has learned a great deal about aphasia in the last century. Because we have this solid data base, our questions and the knowledge resulting from those questions reflect an increasing refinement and sophistication in our theories and our clinical skills. Nevertheless, despite isolated successes and general satisfaction with our efficacy data, we are reluctant to congratulate ourselves because we know how much remains to be done. We also know how many aphasic patients are unable to communicate beyond their very simplest requirements —and some not even that —and we know that many severely and globally aphasic patients are isolated from their families, colleagues, and friends, virtually "prisoners without a language." This book exists because this population exists.

This volume represents an attempt to consolidate what is known about the abilities, the diagnosis, and the treatment of globally aphasic patients from those sources which have contributed to that knowledge. In the first chapter, on the way toward this consolidation, global aphasia is defined from both a theoretical and a practical perspective. The theoretical perspective in that chapter and the chapters that follow is less conspicuous than the practical perspective, which, it is hoped, is prominent throughout this volume. The summary definition is the result of clinically verifiable observations of severely and globally aphasic patients from a number of sources.

Included in the first chapter are brief discussions of lesion size and language deficit, etiology of aphasia, and the role of the right hemisphere in the recovery of language following aphasia, particularly in relation to the globally aphasic patient.

The second chapter is in many ways an extension of the first. As the first chapter suggests, there is some evidence to suppose that severity alone does not adequately differentiate globally aphasic patients from their more fortunate peers. This chapter provides an overview of the evidence which illuminates those differences.

Chapter 3 is an extensive review of assessment in global aphasia. While many of the measures included are appropriate for patients with less severe afflictions, appropriate measures for severely and globally aphasic patients are stressed.

In Chapter 4, patterns of performance on traditional and nontraditional tests for aphasia are used to illustrate the prediction of recovery from aphasia. Included are profiles of typical patients with poor, fair, and good prognoses for recovery.

Chapter 5 is devoted to general considerations in the management of globally aphasic patients. Taken separately, these considerations are neither unique nor novel. They are included here because the combined clinical wisdom inherent in them is potentially such a potent force in treatment.

The specific treatments discussed in Chapter 7 acknowledge that aphasia evolves, and that when it does other treatments may be indicated. When it does not, one or more of the treatments discussed here are at least potentially beneficial. The effects of many of these treatments are discussed in the case illustrations in Chapter 8.

The consolidation attempted in this volume is not unique. It is hoped that it is contemporary, but also that its currency is transient. The globally aphasic patient is deserving of our attention, our research, and our very best clinical endeavors. Through our critical and informed concern, we can ensure that this material has a brief life, and that the globally aphasic patient is the beneficiary of the most robust, sensitive, and effective treatments.

# Chapter 1

# The Nature of the Deficit in Global Aphasia

Alfred North Whitehead once said, "No one has the right to speak more clearly than he thinks." That opinion is unfortunately unenforceable and frequently violated, but most of us have the good fortune to communicate at least as clearly as we think. People suffering from aphasia have literally lost that ability, and the impact is even more devastating in global aphasia. The effect of loss of the ability to speak is an isolation of the person's thoughts and experiences, but there is considerable evidence to suggest that the individual's memories are not lost despite deficits in communication. There is also support for the notion that thought and speech are not inextricably related. The globally aphasic patient seems to know a great deal, thoughts that he or she can share with us only with the greatest difficulty. These patients cannot enlighten us or correct us unless we establish the conditions that allow them to do so. Their thoughts and experiences remain entombed, but the most persistent and patient clinicians will share in a few of their secrets.

Clinicians are not sanguine about those untold secrets or about our frequent failure to elicit them. They have treated, prodded, and tested their patients and touched the boundaries of their own as well as their patients' endurance. They have a few successes and a few failures but no single technique that unfailingly rewards both clinicians and patients. As clinicians, we seem to be armed with only a battery of unfocused, mostly untested clinical techniques. Some of them are more powerful than others, and some focused combinations are even more powerful. In this book, an attempt is made to identify and extol those techniques that are efficacious and separate them from those that are not. The author will also try to identify those patients whose deficits and residual abilities lend themselves to particular treatments.

The ultimate goal of clinicians is to enable globally aphasic patients to share at least some of their experiences and to restore a measure of communicative equilibrium. That noble challenge, however, is continually assaulted by evidence and arguments suggesting that clinicians are powerless to change that communicative impotence. They are told that the deficits in global aphasia are profound, that the prognosis is dim, and that treatment is of little value. This attitude of therapeutic nihilism has been extant for years, and it continues to plague us. The discussion by Schuell, Jenkins, and Jimenez-Pabon (1964) of treatment effects in their Group Five, Irreversible Aphasic Syndrome patients is probably representative of the prevailing attitude: "A bed occupied by a patient who cannot benefit from treatment cannot be occupied by any other patient. The time a clinician spends with a patient who is making no significant gains cannot be spent with another who might" (p. 303). Cohen (1968) stated that "in milder cases of aphasia, the use of speech therapy undoubtedly hastens the patient's recovery, but for patients with severe aphasia, reassurance and psychologic support are probably the major benefits. Therapy appears to be of little value for patients with severe global aphasia, who can neither speak nor understand." At some level, that opinion is perhaps defensible. Clinical time is expensive, the treatment is often drudgery, the rewards are minimal, and the changes are too few and too small.

This attitude will continue to prevail and will continue to influence the attitudes of others who approve or disapprove payment for our efforts until clinicians can demonstrate therapy's benefits. It will not influence the optimistic attitudes of loved ones who share the optimism of the clinicians and may know better than they the effect of treatment. Clinicians can demonstrate their effectiveness by applying treatment appropriately to appropriate patients, by demonstrating that they can apply treatments differentially, by demonstrating that they know the difference between a plateau and a plaint, and by their assurances that their criteria for termination of that treatment are thoughtful, realistic, and humane.

## INCIDENCE AND PREVALENCE OF GLOBAL APHASIA

The incidence of stroke in the general population has been estimated at from 1.7 per 1000 to 2.3 per 1000 (Held, 1975; National Institutes of Health, 1969). This figure increases dramatically as age increases, and there are approximately 2.5 million people suffering from the effects of cerebrovascular accident at any one time (Stein, 1981). The most conservative estimate of aphasic sequelae following stroke is 20 percent, or approximately 50,000 to 100,000 new aphasic patients each year (NIH, 1969). The prevalence of aphasia following stroke is roughly 400,000 to 600,000. The economic impact of stroke, including rehabilitation efforts, is enormous and has been estimated at $10 billion annually (Stein, 1981).

The incidence of global aphasia is difficult to determine. On the basis of figures reported, sometimes anecdotally, the best guess is that from 10 to 30 percent of aphasic patients are globally aphasic, suggesting a globally aphasic population of from 40,000 to 120,000, but Poeck, de Bleser, and Graf von Keyserlingk (1984a) reported that global aphasia is the most common and stable of the major aphasic subtypes. Questioning these actuarial figures is a little like asking what happens to your lap when you stand up, however. The most likely answer is that how "lap" is defined depends on the person's perspective in time. The prevalence of global aphasia too is tied to the temporal domain, but it also depends on the clinician's measurement tools and approach to aphasia, diagnosis, and treatment.


## DEFINING GLOBAL APHASIA

This chapter begins with a traditional definition of aphasia to establish some trail markers and provide us with a basis for a discussion of the ways in which global aphasia differs. Persistent, unremitting global aphasia, in the author's view, is not necessarily just a more severe form of aphasia. Language is impaired, as it is in other forms of aphasia, but one of the things that seem to make global aphasia different from other aphasias is that it seems to be all but immune to traditional forms of therapeutic intervention. If this is true, clinicians, instead of beginning by defining and diagnosing, might simply begin treatment and, when it does not work, base our diagnosis on response to treatment. Despite the logical appeal of such a procedure, too often a patient's failure to respond to traditional treatment draws a curtain across the clinician's therapeutic vision and prevents him or her from expanding the repertoire of treatment techniques. What the patient's failure to improve should suggest is that rather than assuming the patient is untreatable, clinicians should become more innovative and better clinical researchers. The most compelling reasons for us to do so concern the needs of globally aphasic people.

## Traditional Definitions of Aphasia

This book begins with definitions of global aphasia because these definitions help refine treatment focus and stimulate the clinician to think more about what globally aphasic people can do and what they might do. Traditional definitions do not adequately reflect the uniqueness of globally aphasic people, but they provide clinicians with therapeutic baselines for clinicial endeavors. These definitions should not be immune to alterations mandated by time, experience, and evidence. When confronted with new evidence or solid theoretical constructs, however, clinicians may abandon their original operational definitions, but only after testing them for signs of stress, or fracture, or crumbling.

Davis (1982) defines aphasia as "an acquired impairment of language processes underlying receptive and expressive modalities and caused by damage to areas of the brain which are primarily responsible for the language function" (p. 1). To make that definition more germane to global aphasia, it might be possible to simply add a few adjectives and say that aphasia is an acquired, severe impairment of language processes underlying receptive and expressive modalities and caused by extensive damage to areas of the brain that are primarily responsible for the language function.

There are several disadvantages to this conceptual framework. First, such a revision of Davis's definition slights or neglects the nonverbal limitations imposed by global aphasia. Second, it only suggests—and that by inference—a prognosis for the nonverbal limitations imposed by global aphasia. Third, it has limited power to suggest the influence of cognitive abilities in recovery of communication. Fourth, it tells little about what residual skills the globally aphasic patient retains. Finally, because of its popular usage, it may condemn a patient to minimal treatment or no treatment at all. A more comprehensive definition, and one that eliminates some of these disadvantages, was proposed by Goodglass and Kaplan (1983):

> In global aphasia, all aspects of language are so severely impaired that there is no longer a distinctive pattern of preserved versus impaired components. It is only articulation that is sometimes well preserved in the few words or stereotyped utterances that are preserved. Other patients with global aphasia may be totally unable to produce speech sounds voluntarily, even though they may utter an occasional word or short phrase as a spontaneous comment. It may be impossible to complete the Rating Scale Profile of Speech Characteristics for patients with global aphasia, if they do not produce enough speech to rate Melodic Line, Grammatical Form, or Word Finding. Global aphasics sometimes produce stereotyped utterances that may consist of real or nonsense words. Some patients produce a continuous output of syllables that employ a limited set of vowel-consonant combinations and that make no sense, even though they are uttered with

expressive intonation. As noted earlier, such output does not constitute paraphasias. A few special observations on global aphasia are significant. Auditory comprehension of conversation concerning material of immediate personal relevance may appear fairly good in comparison to the patient's poor performance on all the formal auditory comprehension subtests. That is, the patient may indicate "yes" or "no" correctly and with assurance in response to questions about family members, current medical problems, or recent personal events in the hospital or at home. We have also found that many of these patients have a remarkably well-preserved ability to understand geographic place names and locate them. (p. 97)

## An Amended Definition of Global Aphasia

Goodglass and Kaplan's definition just cited (1983) reveals more of the strengths and weaknesses of the globally aphasic patient. Perhaps an even more useful definition is one that is responsive to the temporal domain. An adequate definition should recognize that some patients will improve more rapidly that the clinician's assessments can document. These patients will leave their tremendous deficits behind and move outside the range of global aphasia. They may present initial symptoms that are characteristic of the globally aphasic patient, but after a period of months or years will evolve toward another distinct subtype of aphasia. The last group, fortunately smaller in number, is left with profound deficits that will persist in all modalities despite the healing effects of time. That is not to say that patients in this last group do not evolve. They do, provided their medical and neurologic course does not deteriorate. Their profound deficits persist, however, and they never, at any stage in recovery, demonstrate the promise of their more fortunate compatriots.

The interaction of a number of behavioral and biologic variables, including age, general health, premorbid cognitive status, lesion size and location, and etiology, ensure that few globally aphasic patients will present identical profiles even in the acute stage. In our experience, there seem to be three general categories of globally aphasic patients: acute, evolutional, and chronic. This triad should suggest that global aphasia is more often dynamic than static.

Clinicians are skilled at identifying patients in all three categories even though the distant effects of that severe trauma temporarily blur subtype distinctions. Many patients, perhaps the majority, present global deficits initially. The author has little difficulty agreeing with the neurologist who defines "global" aphasia as severe deficits in expression and reception describing a patient close to onset of the condition. The sine qua non of our profession, however, should be the skill to predict which patients will still have global aphasia at time of discharge. Such a judgment is frequently based on intuition and data, that peculiar mix of skills common to professions. If the profession is to evolve, these decisions must move from clinical biases and generalities to data-based probabilities. As a first step toward that goal, the author proposes this definition:

> Global aphasia is a severe, acquired impairment of communicative ability across all language modalities, and often no single communicative modality is strikingly better than another. Visual nonverbal problem-solving abilities are often severely depressed as well and are usually compatible with language performance. It usually results from extensive damage to the language zones of the left hemisphere but may result from smaller, subcortical lesions. In general, the smaller the lesion and the greater its distance from primary language zones, the greater the potential for recovery. Prognosis is frequently predicated on variability of performance in the early stages of recovery. The acute stage of recovery generally does not exceed two to seven days unless other physiological factors intervene but may continue far beyond that time. Variability much beyond this time suggests an evolutional global aphasia. Extremely limited variability usually suggests that a chronic global aphasia will emerge.

## LESION SIZE AND LANGUAGE DEFICIT

Although there is not an unvaryingly high correlation of lesion size with language deficit, the relationship is very strong. It is probably the single most critical factor in failure to recover.

According to Goodglass (1981), global aphasia is usually associated with a large perisylvian lesion involving the frontal, temporal, and parietal lobes. This area is supplied by the middle cerebral artery. It is the most frequent circulatory subsystem involved in left hemisphere cerebrovascular accident. As shown in Figure 1-1, the middle cerebral artery provides nourishment to a relatively large area of the cerebral cortex.

The relationship of large lesions to severe language deficits is traditional. This relationship has been supported by Kertesz (1979), among others, who found a positive, statistically significant correlation between recovery of comprehension and lesion size. Although he noted "remarkable" recovery of comprehension of some globally aphasic patients with large middle cerebral artery lesions, Wernicke's area was usually spared in these patients. Kertesz's findings supported the clinician's insight that "the larger the lesion, the less the recovery," but he cautioned that in individual cases, a critically placed lesion could produce a severe, persisting aphasia.

Selnes, Niccum, and Rubens (1982) found that those patients who demonstrated little or no recovery of auditory comprehension had lesions involving the posterior superior temporal lobe that frequently extended

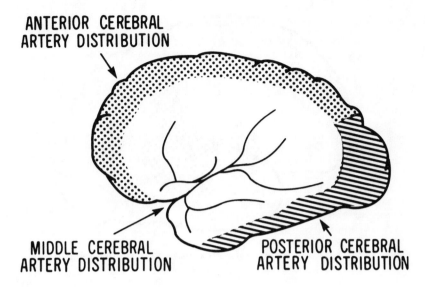

**ANTERIOR CEREBRAL ARTERY DISTRIBUTION**

**MIDDLE CEREBRAL ARTERY DISTRIBUTION**

**POSTERIOR CEREBRAL ARTERY DISTRIBUTION**

**Figure 1–1.** Distribution of the middle cerebral artery.

into the supramarginal gyrus. Lesion volume in these patients ranged from 60 cm³ to 183 cm³, with a mean volume of 116 cm³. When the posterior superior temporal lobe was spared, recovery was greater, and the majority of that recovery occurred prior to 3 months post onset. This finding is in distinct contrast to that for patients with posterior superior temporal lobe involvement, who recovered much more gradually. Those patients whose auditory comprehension and nonverbal performance improved most by 6 months post onset had the smallest lesions (4 to 47 cm³) and the lowest frequency of posterior superior temporal lobe and supramarginal gyrus involvement (1 of 12). Those patients who improved least had the largest lesions (60 to 183 cm³) and the most frequent occurrence of posterior superior temporal lobe (7 of 7) and superior marginal gyrus involvement (6 of 7). Figure 1–2 shows a composite of cerebral cortex involvement in global aphasia from a lateral view.

Figure 1–3 is a schematic representation of a computed tomographic (CT) template in global aphasia showing a typical lesion in the coronal plane.

Larger lesions usually produce major deficits, but lesions of similar size do not always produce similarly severe deficits. There is also intriguing evidence to suggest that at least some cases of global aphasia may be produced by a large, totally subcortical lesion of the capsular striatal zone (Poeck et al., 1984b). Other subcortical structures that have been implicated in other aphasic subtypes include the insula, thalamus, caudate and lenticular nuclei, putamen, globus pallidus, and white matter

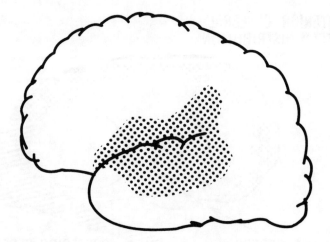

**Figure 1–2.** Area of the cerebral cortex involved in global aphasia.

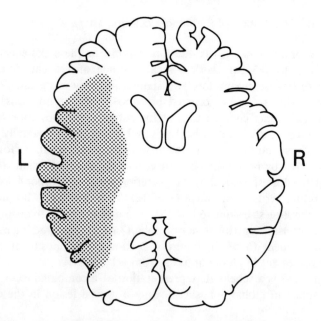

**Figure 1-3.** Schematic drawing of a computed tomographic (CT) scan in global aphasia.

subserving the frontal, temporal, and parietal lobes. It has not been suggested that global aphasia may result from damage to these structures, but it is at least theoretically possible that significant damage to one or more of them could result in significant deficits.

The data of Poeck and colleagues are potentially very important clinically because, since the corpus callosum and striatum seem to be more involved in the transmission of signals than in the formulation of signals, perhaps this particular "global" aphasia is primarily *motor* in nature. If this is true, failure to demonstrate comprehension may be caused by an inability to perform volitional oral or gestural movements despite the absence of peripheral weakness or paralysis. If that is the case, the descriptive term "aphasia" is a misnomer.

Benson (1979) has also reported that a single infarct along the sylvian lips with few neighborhood signs will produce a devastating aphasia.

It is beyond the scope of this chapter to discuss the frequency of occurrence or the mechanisms involved in language deficits created by subcortical lesions. The issue is complicated and controversial, and the interested reader should best examine selected readings. In summary, however, it is safe to say that in general the larger the lesion the poorer the eventual outcome. This is particularly true if the lesion is greater than 60 cm$^3$ and involves the frontal, temporal, and parietal language zones, and particularly the posterior temporal gyrus. Small, strategically placed lesions can, however, produce a severe, persisting aphasia. It is not known in what manner the recovery curves for these patients differ from those with aphasia caused by large lesions with foci in Broca's and Wernicke's areas.

## ETIOLOGY

Global aphasia is most frequently produced when both the anterior (Broca's) and posterior (Wernicke's) language areas are destroyed or dysfunctional. Because these two areas are supplied by separate branches of the MCA (pre-rolandic and middle temporal) global aphasia is usually produced by an arterial trunk occlusion resulting in a large perisylvian infarct.

The cause of global aphasia is usually thrombotic rather than embolic. This distinction is critical in the medical management of stroke and may be equally important in eventual language recovery.

Different causes produce different effects on recovery (Porch, 1981). Patients suffering from hemorrhage, trauma, and thromboembolic episodes generally have emphatically different recovery curves. The least impressive of these is the recovery curve for thromboembolic strokes. The term "thromboembolic" is a concession to the difficulty of differentiating thrombotic episodes from embolic episodes, but embolic episodes may be more frequent than previously thought. A report by Van Horn and Hawes, 1982, for example, described three cases of global aphasia that resulted from two discrete lesions stemming from an embolic encephalopathy.

## THE SEQUELAE OF GLOBAL APHASIA

Because the lesion is usually so large, associated sequelae are common. These include right hemiparesis or hemiplegia, right-sided sensory loss, and right homonymous hemianopsia. Oral, nonverbal apraxia, apraxia of speech, limb apraxia, and constructional apraxia are thought to be frequent residual deficits, but their presence is more difficult to determine. Adequate tests that do not require verbal mediation are not available.

Hemi-inattention, or hemineglect, is also frequently associated with global aphasia. The term refers to a variety of behaviors, principally a lack of response to sensory stimuli delivered to one side of the body, sensory and motor neglect of one side of the individual's body and extrapersonal space, and verbal denial of illness or hemiplegia. Apparently more common in right-sided lesions, it is generally thought to last only a few days to several weeks. Its existence in aphasia is controversial; some authorities believe that left hemisphere lesions resulting in aphasia render the patient unable to understand or complete tests or to produce speech that might reveal inattention characteristics. Others support a right hemisphere predominance for these deficits but do not deny the possibility of hemineglect caused by dominant hemisphere lesions.

Apraxia is the impairment of ability to perform practiced, volitional movements in the relative absence of paralysis, paresis, incoordination, or comprehension deficit. The relationship of apraxia to aphasia appears to be a strong one, but not all authors have been convincing in demonstrating the strength of the relationship. Goodglass (1981) did not find a significant correlation between the appearance of apraxia and severity, and Alajouanine and Lhermitte (1960) found no direct relationship between apraxia and aphasia. Kertesz (1984b), however, studied the frequency of apraxia in a large number of aphasic and nonaphasic individuals. He found a very strong association between the two disorders. The most general finding of this study was that there is a hierarchical impairment of gesture—attributable to apraxia, which is related to severity of aphasia—and type of aphasia. Globally aphasic patients were most frequently apractic, and lesion size and gestural impairment were significantly related, in both the acute (less than 45 days post onset) and the chronic stages (greater than 330 days post onset). In this study, lesion size was split into two groups: small lesions were those that constituted less than 10 percent of hemispheric volume, and large lesions were those that made up more than one third of hemispheric volume. Nevertheless,

18 percent of patients in the acute group who had large lesions, and 30 percent of the patients in the chronic group who had large lesions, were not apractic.

One implication of this study is that those patients with the most severe aphasia, and the largest lesions, may be prevented from displaying what competence remains when gestural or verbal responses are required in the early stages of recovery. Recovery of praxis is reported (Kertesz, 1984a) to roughly parallel recovery of language for most aphasic patients, but Kertesz found that recovery from apraxia is more pronounced in the early stages of recovery. This finding may also explain in part the paradoxical recovery patterns for globally aphasic patients reported by Sarno and Levita (1981), who found greater recovery after 6 months post onset.

A second implication is that gestural abilities in global aphasia, which may be resistant to treatment because they are physiologically based, may deserve greater attention in later stages of recovery than in earlier stages. This implication may also contribute to our understanding of initial failure to respond to traditional treatments and striking response to nontraditional treatments—for example, Visual Action Therapy (VAT)—in the later stages of recovery.

## THE RIGHT HEMISPHERE'S ROLE IN RECOVERY OF LANGUAGE FOLLOWING APHASIA

The right hemisphere is an appealing candidate on which to rely for the resumption of speech and language activities following damage to left hemisphere (usually the dominant, verbal hemisphere). The right hemisphere is similar in size, weight, configuration, and structure to the left hemisphere (Geschwind and Levitsky, 1968). Perhaps because it appears to be intact in patients with global aphasia, it is frequently implicated as at least the potential source of language ability in aphasic patients. The evidence cited to support this argument is persuasive. Hemispherectomy and callosal lesion studies, for example, in both infants and adults have demonstrated that individuals with functioning right hemispheres are capable of acquiring language when the dominant hemisphere is absent or disconnected from the rest of the brain. Hemispherectomy studies, particularly those reported for children, have frequently been cited as support for the right hemisphere's abilities (Gazzaniga, 1971; Sperry, 1968). A study by Day and Ulatowska (1978) disturbs our data-based complacency. These authors reported that although language eventually emerges in children hemispherectomized at an early age, it does not develop as fully or at the same rate as in these children's peers. This suggests that, for whatever reason, the right hemisphere may not be the linguistic equal of the left hemisphere to begin with.

An additional barrier, age, is also placed on the right hemisphere. The ability of the right hemisphere to respond to novel stimuli decreases substantially with increasing age (Lenneberg, 1967). It might be assumed, from Lenneberg's evidence and that of others, that establishing laterality is a more potent deterrent than age. According to Lenneberg, for example, handedness is generally established by 8 years of age—in extreme cases by 12 years—and the likelihood of reacquiring language after dominant hemispherectomy decreases substantially after that.

People in general are reluctant to assume that they become *unable* to perform a task simply because they get old. They would rather believe that they only become less proficient, or that it takes them longer to learn a new task. Few would accept graciously the notion that age diminishes their potential so drastically. Perhaps it does not. The debate continues sporadically by learned authorities in scholarly journals, whose data are sometimes distorted by the popular press. Some of the basic premises and, it is hoped, the flavor of both sides of that debate are presented here.

Jaynes (1976) has said that the "minor" hemisphere once communicated with the gods.

Searleman (1977) has summarized more substantial evidence and scientific data in support of the right hemisphere, taken from a variety of sources and an impressive collection of data:

1. A healthy right hemisphere can take over some language functions following left hemisphere damage, because
   a. Aphasic persons who have recovered some language functioning lose this if the right hemisphere is destroyed.
   b. Aphasic individuals who have some residual speech retain this during left hemisphere injection in a Wada test.
   c. Some aphasic persons have a left ear advantage on dichotic listening tests and some have a left visual field advantage on tachistoscopic tests (but none were tested premorbidly).

Searleman concluded that sensory field preference for verbal stimuli shifts direction in favor of the right hemisphere following damage to the left.

Despite the impressive phalanx of support, this theory of right hemisphere capacity to develop has its detractors. Moscovitch (1981), who has marshaled a substantial body of evidence on his own, says

> A great many patients with damage to the left hemisphere are often profoundly aphasic, alexic, or word-deaf despite having a healthy, intact right hemisphere. This fact alone should dispel the view that the extensive linguistic skills of the right hemisphere, found in some split brain patients,

also typify the performance of the right hemisphere of most people. Either there are large individual differences or the right hemisphere of many patients is prevented from displaying its skills even when they are most needed. (p. 49)

It has been known for some time that there is considerable variability within and among the cerebral hemispheres for the localization of function (Ojeman, 1978, 1979). A relatively recent study has demonstrated what appears to be an inequality in the right hemispheres of some globally aphasic patients. Pieniadz, Naeser, Koff, and Levine (1983) examined cerebral hemispheric measurements in normal subjects and patients with global aphasia. They found that there are atypical cerebral hemispheric asymmetries among right-handers and suggested that these hemispheric differences may be associated with superior recovery on the one-word level in comprehension, repetition, and naming. These atypical hemispheric asymmetries include a larger right occipital region, a longer, lower, more horizontally oriented right sylvian fissure and a larger right planum temporale. In the left hemisphere these anatomical areas are assumed to be substrates for language processing. It may be reasonable, therefore, to postulate that the atypical, asymmetrical appearance of the right hemisphere may signify some anomalous language dominance.

If the right hemisphere fails in many patients, it could be that this failure results from too small a lesion in the left. Moscovitch (1981) has suggested that a substantial portion of the left hemisphere must be incapacitated before the right hemisphere can be freed to participate. Although no one has seriously suggested left hemispherectomy as a treatment for global aphasia, it is conceivable that only near-total destruction or removal of the incapacitated left hemisphere frees the right hemisphere. Nevertheless, very large lesions do not, in fact, seem to free the right hemisphere unless the language capabilities of that hemisphere are less significant than believed.

Dennis (1980), has said

> at best, the isolated right hemisphere can analyze the lexical and grammatical morphemic structure of the sentence and, as a result, can find the conceptual or logical meaning of simple passive sentences. It is only the left hemisphere that has available to it the strategy of integrating rules with surface structure syntax to derive meaning. (p. 43)

Despite popularized media attention to hemispheric differences there is, according to Sperry (1984), no evidence that this can be done. He has eloquently and coherently summarized the evidence:

> the experimentally observed polarity in right-left cognitive style is an idea in general with which it is very easy to run wild. You can read today that things such as intuition, the seat of the subconscious, creativity, paraphy-

sic sensitivity, the mind of the Orient, ethnocultural disposition, hypnotic susceptibility, the roots of counter-culture, altered states of consciousness—and whatnot—all reside predominantly in the right hemisphere. The extent to which extrapolations of this kind may eventually prove to be more fact or fancy will require many years to determine. Meantime it is important to remember that the two hemispheres in the normal intact brain tend regularly to function closely together as a unit and that different states of mind are apt to involve different hierarchical and organizational levels or front-back and other differentiations as well as differences in laterality. (p. 668)

More data are needed, and these data are being collected. Positron emission tomography (PET) and Magnetic Resonance Imaging (MRI) for example, which permit dynamic, functional assessment of brain activity, are significant advances in our understanding of these mechanisms and their differences. It is conceivable that they will eventually be an equal partner with the clinician's intuition.

## SUMMARY

The factors discussed in the previous section are important to an understanding of the nature of global aphasia and to the treatment of its deficits. Although the data base is inadequate and speculation has fueled controversy, it seems likely that the right hemisphere is only potentially a powerful ally in treatment. An uncontested role for the right hemisphere in speech and language recovery is still not tenable despite the evidence and opinion favoring its participation.

The data summarized here are not conclusively in favor of one position over another. They do, however, suggest an unattractive conclusion: that lesions of any magnitude that do not resolve may interfere with right hemisphere involvement in the reacquisition of language. Furthermore, the right hemisphere, as much as we appreciate its unique qualities, at its best may be capable of only the most elementary linguistic operations. These operations favor comprehension but also may include repetition and naming. Finally, damage to the left hemisphere may suppress even those poor abilities.

It has also been seen that there is general agreement concerning several parameters in global aphasia. First, an attitude of therapeutic nihilism has prevailed for years. The unwillingness of some clinicians to provide services, and a reluctance on the part of funding sources to support these services, is a reflection of this attitude. This pessimism is a response to the staggering size of the lesion, the residual sequelae, which are difficult to identify or circumvent, and the resistance of global aphasia to traditional therapeutic intervention.

Given this evidence, optimism, mixed with an appreciation of reality and a reluctance to accept the inevitable, may be as important an asset to the clinician as his or her professional affiliation or library. Despite the ponderous weight of the negative evidence, we have reasons for optimism. In succeeding sections of this book, these reasons may become clearer.

# Chapter 2

# Physiological Recovery and Behavioral Sequelae in Global Aphasia

This section begins with a discussion of mechanisms potentially involved in the suppression of language in aphasia, particularly in global aphasia. They may explain in part why recovery patterns in global aphasia differ from those seen in less severe forms.

## PHYSIOLOGY OF RECOVERY

Diaschisis, first described by von Monakow in 1914 (cited in Rubens, 1977) is defined as the decreased responsiveness and dysfunction of intact neurons remote from the damaged area following brain damage. According to some authors (Meyer et al., 1971; Smith, 1972), that definition may be too limiting. They would also include the temporary suspension of functions of intact ipsilateral or contralateral hemispheric structures remote from the focal lesion.

Riese (1970) emphasized the importance of the "momentum" of the lesion and the "distance effects" as confounding factors in the cerebral localization of language and other functions. Smith (1972) in fact suggested that the association of severe impairment of *language* and *nonlanguage* functions "reflects either the presence of associated right hemisphere lesions or radiation of effects of irritative left sided lesions that may inhibit language or nonlanguage functions of the right hemisphere" (p. 200). Given this hypothesis, it is conceivable that the verbal and nonverbal deficits seen in global aphasia may be due in part to diaschisis and its remote effects, which attenuate performance by the right hemisphere or other intact structures. Meyer and colleagues (1971) found that the duration and severity of diaschisis increased with the magnitude of the infarction, and they also suggested that diaschisis is more severe and lasts longer in older patients with acute unilateral cerebral infarctions.

Meyer and colleagues (1971) also suggested that diaschisis may be associated with bilateral reduction of blood flow following cerebral infarction. They say that this reduction of blood flow occurs frequently in unilateral cerebral infarcts and approaches normal values again in the *healthy* hemisphere *only* in younger patients (under 59 years of age) and then only after months or even years. In older patients (over 60 years) hemispheric blood flow in the healthy hemisphere may never return to normal values. Meyer and associates observed that regional cerebral blood flow (RCBF) was depressed in both hemispheres during the first 3 weeks following lateralized cerebral infarctions. After that time they noted that the depression of cerebral blood flow in both hemispheres increased significantly in the unaffected, healthy hemispheres. This was particularly true of younger patients.

Finally, Meyer and colleagues (1971) reported that blood flow correlated with the magnitude of lesion, and they emphasized that the return of adequate collateral circulation was the single most important factor in recovery from cerebral ischemia.

This concept is theoretically important to an understanding of global aphasia, the paradoxical recovery patterns reported by Sarno and Levita (1981), and possible right hemisphere involvement in the acquisition, maintenance, and recovery of language.

## BEHAVIORAL CHANGES AND INTELLECT IN GLOBAL APHASIA

McNeil (1982) offered a definition of aphasia that goes beyond traditional definitions. It is offered here because of its forthright hypotheses to account for deficits that may be involved in global aphasia:

Aphasia is a multimodality physiological inefficiency with *greater than loss* of verbal symbolic manipulations (e.g., association, storage, retrieval, and rule implementation). In isolated form, it is caused by focal damage to cortical and/or subcortical structures of the hemisphere(s) dominant for such symbolic manipulations. It is affected by and affects other physiological, information processing, and cognitive processes to the degree that they support, interact with, or are supported by the verbal symbolic deficits. (p. 693) (italics added)

One of the more important elements in that definition is the linking of verbal symbolic deficits (language) with cognitive processes. That notion is not new or unique. Wepman (1972), for example, proposed that the deficits seen in aphasia may result not from a linguistic deficit but from a thought process deficit. In his view, aphasia may affect people differently depending on whether the impairment lies in the inability to have and maintain "thoughts" separately from the ability to formulate verbal symbols related to these thoughts. If the "thoughts" are intact in aphasia, the implications are that (1) cognitive processes, including general intelligence, memory processes, and, possibly, attention, are intact, and (2) aphasia is more a deficit in performance than a deficit in competence because the "idea," or "thought," would appear to require verbal mediation, even for its internalized appearance.

McNeil (1982) summarized the evidence to support a performance deficit in opposition to a competence deficit in aphasia. In his view, aphasia can be thought of as an inefficient, fluctuating biological system. For evidence, he cites that fact that aphasia can be transient and that transient aphasia cannot be differentiated from more permanent forms. He concludes that a temporary inefficiency or interfering condition must therefore account for the performance deficit. For example, the language deficits seen in the early stages of recovery in a patient with evolving Broca's aphasia may resemble those seen in a patient whose aphasia evolves (improves) to Broca's. One implication of the foregoing example is that aphasia is dynamic and that, in the early stages, labels might best be withheld until the deficits stabilize. Another is the suggestion that aphasia is not primarily, or permanently, a loss of language.

McNeil (1982) also cited evidence from the performance of aphasic patients on an auditory comprehension task. In this task, patients demonstrated variable ability on equally difficult tasks they could sometimes perform adequately, but not consistently. McNeil postulated that some "internally generated oscillator" controlling attention and resource allocation might account for these inconsistent deficits.

McNeil (1982) viewed the stimulability of the aphasic patient as evidence that the basic units of language are not lost. Manipulation of stimulus characteristics and conditions improves or diminishes performance, suggesting that at least some language is intact, and that certain stimulus conditions demonstrate that aphasic individuals can intuit the rules and structures of language, although they cannot readily use them.

McNeil's evidence (1982) was based primarily on the study of aphasias in which some preserved performance can be elicited (that is, in more moderate to mild aphasia or distinct aphasic subtypes). The apparent reluctance of McNeil and others to include globally aphasic patients in these studies suggests a tacit assumption that globally aphasic patients are different or that there is a loss of *both* competence and performance. Perhaps this is so. The difficult of eliciting interpretable responses from globally aphasic patients, however, presents a significant barrier to penetrating studies. Perseveration, apraxia, severity, and inability to attend conspire to prevent assessment of diminished competence above a recognition level.

Despite these deficits, there is no reason to believe that lesions of greater than 40 cm$^3$ suddenly deprive a patient of his or her linguistic competence and cognitive processes but slightly smaller lesions do not. It is possible to demonstrate that the patients with such lesions have memories and can think about them at some level, and it can be demonstrated that the patient has this capacity, provided that the stimulus conditions are right and the clinician assumes most of the burden of communication. It is known that patients' abilities vary, that patients are stimulable, and that they can intuit linguistic structures and rules. They can distinguish sense from nonsense, home from the hospital, and a Lambourghini from a Lotus, but the conclusive demonstration of this competence has so far proved to be elusive. There are no tests that allow the clinician to circumvent these barriers and release the "prisoner without a language" Conniff (1983). What evidence is available is mostly anecdotal or results from tests that may have been applied and interpreted inappropriately.

## LANGUAGE, INTELLECT, AND CEREBRAL DOMINANCE

Davis (1982) has stated that "most of us possess two modes of cognitive activity that are separated by the cerebral commissure." These modes are described as (1) analytic, rational, logical, and verbal, for the left hemisphere, and (2) holistic, intuitive, emotional and spatial, for the right hemisphere (p. 66). Are these traits truly so dichotomized? Some authors think not. Smith (1972), for example, found impairment in nonlanguage reasoning capacities to be associated more frequently with severe comprehension deficits than with moderate or slight comprehension deficits, and Marie (1906) thought that persons who incurred brain damage associated with aphasia always showed some degree of impairment in language competence as well as some degree of intellectual impairment. Nevertheless, the evidence (Lebrun and Hoops, 1974; Wertz et al., 1981; Zangwill, 1960) suggests that there is no significant correlation between nonverbal problem-solving ability and language ability. This failure to demonstrate a relationship may depend on the nonverbal task.

The most widely used measure of nonverbal reasoning in normal and pathologic groups is Raven's *Coloured Progressive Matrices (RCPM)* (Raven, 1962). On the basis of this test, few studies have demonstrated a consistent relationship between severity of aphasia and nonverbal reasoning (e.g., Wertz et al., 1981). When severity of language is controlled, however, a relatively consistent relationship emerges. Collins (1982), for example, found a significant, positive correlation ($r = .69$, $p < .05$) between language ability, as measured by the *Porch Index of Communicative Ability (PICA)* (Porch, 1967) and performance on the RCPM by globally aphasic patients in the early stages of recovery. Surprisingly, this deficit does not endure, and in time it approaches values obtained for patients with moderate to mild aphasia.

Because the right hemisphere appears to contribute significantly to nonverbal reasoning tasks, this ability would be expected to remain relatively unimpaired in left hemisphere lesions. As has been seen, however, there is some reason to suspect that the right hemisphere's ability is impaired following lesions resulting in aphasia. Most globally aphasic patients score between 0 and 20 on the RCPM in the early stages of recovery, but performance rarely remains at that level. Improvement usually occurs sometime after 6 months have elapsed from onset. There is no adequate explanation for this paradoxical recovery. One hypothesis is that this recovery is unrelated to treatment and may be predicted on physiological recovery, reversible disaschisis, and a physiological "readiness" period. In addition, the deficits seen in global aphasia on lower level tasks, such as copying and matching, are thought by some to be signs of bilateral brain damage (Porch, personal communication, 1982). There is additional evidence to suggest that these deficits in nonverbal problem solving are not permanent, and that it is not uncommon for significant improvement to continue for years, or for patients to make dramatic gains in these abilities after the period of spontaneous recovery has passed.

## COMPREHENSION AND RECOGNITION IN THE GLOBALLY APHASIC PATIENT

Comprehension seems to operate at different levels, ranging from a relatively superficial grasp of meaning to a deep, detailed understanding (Paivio and Begg, 1981). These authors stated that "our scientific understanding of the nature of comprehension is itself still relatively superficial and primitive" (p. 169). So, too, unfortunately, is our grasp of comprehension in global aphasia. Because globally aphasic patients are unable to respond verbally, they are judged unable to understand. Yet they appear to *recognize* at a level very near that of other, less severely involved patients. This is inferred because they can demonstrate it. It is not yet known how far comprehension extends beyond that, or how best to test for it. One potentially useful model is the classical conditioning paradigm. Collins and Wertz (1974) attempted to assess comprehension in aphasic patients using this paradigm. In this study, the conditioned stimuli were verbal and nonverbal pictorial and lexical stimuli. The hypothesis was that if comprehension were intact but could not be adequately demonstrated by conventional measurement, perhaps conditioning an autonomic response, the eyeblink, to presentations of verbal (auditory and lexical) matches and mismatches would tap that ability. The results of the study were inconclusive but potentially useful.

The globally aphasic patient can match single words from several foils at a level much greater than that predicted by chance; match pictures and objects; indicate wrong words from a list of misspelled words; and recognize pictures of familiar places, objects, faces, and brand names. Also, they can mark appropriate locations on an outline map and in a picture of a room filled with familiar objects (Wapner and Gardner, 1979).

Globally aphasic patients can often follow whole body commands (e.g., "stand up," "sit down") (Goodglass, 1981) and comprehend some personally relevant questions; they can also distinguish between meaningful and meaningless speech and among types of requests (Boller and Green, 1972; Green and Boller, 1974) and identify familiar environmental sounds (Spinnler and Vignolo, 1966). They likewise recognize familiar faces, voices, places, and melodies, and often recognize humor, metaphor, and absurdities, responding appropriately and consistently if not accurately. Wallace and Canter (1984) have even found that severely aphasic patients respond with significantly greater success when presented with personally relevant language materials than with otherwise similar nonpersonal language materials.

Many of these recognition skills are reflections òf learned experience, and one argument for their existence is that they are the product of right hemisphere or subcortical structures. Another is that they do not require a depth of linguistic skill but are somehow supralinguistic, metalinguistic, sublinguistic, or nonlinguistic, or some combination of these. If they require linguistic competence, however minimal, the implication is that this minimal competence can be capitalized on, not just to communicate but also to use language meaningfully and appropriately, and not only for comprehension but also for expression.

## EXPRESSIVE SKILLS

The communicative skills of the globally aphasic patient suggest either a basic, unlateralized communicative competence or competence based on right hemisphere capabilities that seem to be more adept at comprehension than expression. The globally aphasic patient is most impaired in the expressive modalities, and this receptive advantage, as in most other aphasias, continues throughout recovery.

Globally aphasic patients can often imitate single words and some phrases, but speech is rarely functional. As will be seen later, there is probably a small subgroup of aphasic patients whose language production is restricted to the fluent, repetitive production of one consonant-vowel (CV) syllable (deBleser and Poeck, 1984). The general clinical perception is that these patients have good comprehension and are able to convey communicative intentions by means of suprasegmental features. deBleser and Poeck, however, found that these patients have no "language systematic features left." They remarked that the discrepancy between extremely low test scores and the general clinical impression of preserved communicative ability (expressive use of supralinguistic features to express surprise, anger, questioning, and so forth) is a misconception.

The six globally aphasic patients studied by deBleser and Poeck (1984) did not display sufficient prosodic variability to convey communicative intentions by formal test. Is the notion that prosodic proficiency is preserved, commonly held by clinicians and others, a misconception? The author does not think so, but the answer is not known. It may be that formal testing, of the sort done by deBleser and Poeck, does not reflect the ability of these patients to use a single recurring utterance with a variety of inflections to convey intent spontaneously, a finding clinicians report consistently.

Except for their fluent productions of single syllables, the extremely poor performance of these patients places them at the bottom of the distribution for global aphasia. deBleser and Poeck (1984), in fact, argued that globally aphasic patients should be subdivided into standard nonfluent patients, or those who do not produce recurrent utterances, and nonstandard fluent globally aphasic patients, those who do.

Globally aphasic patients may also copy letters and some figures accurately; may learn to write their names and the names of family members; and, with training, may learn approximations of names of family members or words of daily living. But spontaneous, functional writing is sparse or, in many cases, absent. Volitional production of meaningful gestures may be more functional in many globally aphasic patients than writing, but the development of these skills requires extensive training.

## SUMMARY

The evidence cited here, some of it clearly controversial, presents clinicians with a difficult clinical dilemma to which there is as yet no satisfactory solution. On the one hand, there is reason to believe that globally aphasic patients recover differently from other aphasic patients. Improvement may be related to physiological recovery and may produce a persistent suppression of latent skills or inadequate ability to participate in treatment. One implication that cannot be ignored is that treatment may not be beneficial in the early stages of recovery.

On the other hand, under present guidelines, treatment is rarely approved for more than 1 year post onset, and to deny treatment for the first 6 months is to deny the patient the hope of recovery. Rather than await an administrative decision based on inadequate information, it is necessary to collect more and better treatment data, of the quality Sarno and Levita (1979) provided. Clinicians need to know whether early treatment is prophylactic, premature, or problematic. They also need to know if there are individual differences among globally aphasic patients that can be predicted, and by what methods, and they need to know what treatment methods are diversely efficacious.

The brief review of the literature cited here suggests that globally aphasic patients possess minimal linguistic abilities, most of which favor comprehension. In time, patients' cognitive skills appear to approximate those of their less involved aphasic counterparts. To attribute the failure of these patients to perform to their incompetence may be inappropriate and may be the result of inadequate measurement.

Chapter 3 is an attempt to focus measurement of global aphasia so that it reflects not only the patient's deficits but also his or her residual skills. In currently popular jargon, these skills are "can do" behaviors.

# Chapter 3

# Evaluation and Diagnosis

## A PHILOSOPHY OF DIAGNOSIS

An adequate evaluation should tell what a patient can and cannot do, in addition to as much about the "why" as the data can muster. It should provide a profile of impairment, and, with data obtained from other sources, present speculations and hypotheses to be tested. The evaluation should also point to etiology and allow the clinician to compare patients to other patients within a population. Finally, it should allow the clinician to attach a label to that set of symptoms.

Clinicians recognize that aphasia is typically more dynamic than static. They also know that labels are often no more than shorthand and that many patients' symptoms will not fit into any one diagnostic category. They do not treat their patients on the basis of a label. Labels serve a purpose because they communicate; they allow clinicians to talk about patients in a general sense with other professionals. They allow the results of treatment for one patient to be compared with the results for another. Finally, labels are the culmination of a synthesis of data that reflects the professionalism and skills of the clinician. Describing behaviors requires only observation and notation. Knowing what the particular set of symptoms means combines the art and science of diagnosis, and this is the clinician's reward and contribution.

## HYPOTHESIS TESTING

Patient data do not always make sense immediately, particularly if the clinician fails to look beyond the objective evidence. The data begin to make sense when objective findings are mixed with patient histories, family interviews, and medical records. Tentative hypotheses are then formulated about the results. Hypotheses may be based on formal or informal test data and are then tested with supplemental tests or with measures of learning conducted over a session or over several sessions. Hypothesis testing permits the clinician to narrow or expand diagnostic, prognostic, and treatment foci as each hypothesis is tested.

A hypothesis is really a hypothetical question, but it does not have to be—and should not be—a rhetorical one. A hypothesis should be a rational, possible explanation that accounts for a set of facts, and that can be tested by further investigation.

A hypothesis can be as simple as "This patient should benefit from combined auditory and lexical presentation of stimuli." Such a hypothesis can be tested by comparing auditory presentation alone with lexical presentation alone, and each with combined auditory and lexical stimuli. Another hypothesis might be, "This patient is not aphasic. His poor visual acuity makes him incapable of reading fine print," which is then tested with larger print material.

None of the questions these hypotheses raise are trivial, and the answers will have a significant effect on treatment planning. A series of questions, formally or informally stated, and with test conditions carefully controlled, will provide a deeper understanding of the patient and the most effective methods of management. Adequate documentation of both questions and results will provide a deeper understanding of the disorder.

## FORMAL AND INFORMAL MEASURES OF EVALUATION, BASELINE, AND CHANGE

Formal test results permit an understanding of the patient's deficits and skills and allow the clinician to document the effects of treatment, but the information gained from other sources should be valued equally. The order of the elements in the foregoing sentence could be reversed and the intent would be unaltered. Neither assessment can stand alone—informal assessment must inevitably succumb to objectivity, and objective test results must be supplemented with informal assessment and information from other sources.

The clinician needs to know, for example, what conditions might influence performance. These conditions can be tested empirically, as

Marshall and King (1972) did, by examining "order" effects—for example, of morning versus afternoon, of performance before or after other therapies, or of the effect on performance of medication, other testing, or other events. It is necessary to review the patient's progress and condition periodically by reviewing his or her chart frequently, by meeting with staff members, and, equally important, by meeting with family members.

The clinician needs to know about the patient's life before and after the illness. Was he or she depressed, laconic, or energetic? Did the patient stutter? Did he or she have any hobbies and if so, which ones? The assessment is not complete until the chart is reviewed thoroughly, the patient's schedule is examined for potential conflicts or treatment effects, staff members have been consulted, and family and friends have been interviewed.

Not every measure is suitable for every patient, nor is it necessary to administer every test in the clinical repertoire. Ideally, an assessment should *sample* communicative behaviors across a variety of settings and under a variety of stimulus conditions. If the formal assessment does not allow an adequate sampling or include a variety of stimulus conditions, the formal battery should be augmented with informal measures designed to clarify the diagnosis, make the patient feel more at ease, and identify those conditions that enhance performance.

## Informal Assessment

The best informal measures are really attempts to structure and formalize informality. Because they rely on more natural conditions for their data, patients may feel less like they are under scrutiny, and informal assessment, at bedside or in the cafeteria, is an important adjunct to formal assessment. These informal assessments, however, are not substitutes, and to base a diagnosis on subjective data and environmental artifact is a disservice to patients.

## Formal Assessment

Informal assessment—or, better yet, formal assessment disguised as conversation—is advisable when formal assessment is not practical (for example, at bedside or with very sick patients). Formal testing is advocated when possible because major errors are less likely to be made in diagnosis or prognosis. Because the tests are standardized on the aphasic population, clinicians can feel reasonably sure about their results and more secure in their interpretations. Formal tests are anchored in empirical data, usually on very large numbers of patients, and help to give stability to diagnoses and prognoses. Also, because they are standardized, they provide a framework for accountability, allowing clinicians to justify their decisions to treat, to continue treatment, or to discontinue treatment. The very best tests meet these criteria, but knowing when to test is probably as important as knowing which test to use.

## EARLY TESTING AND OTHER MATTERS

Schuell (1965) advised testing when patients were medically stable to obtain meaningful and interpretable results. Most clinicians violate this timetable, and it is unclear whether patients or data suffer for it. It is known that patients' conditions evolve, and the timing of this evolution will vary with size of lesion and a number of other factors. We are indebted to Kertesz (1979) and others for documenting the various forms of evolution in aphasia. Clinicians know that their treatment focus will shift as the aphasia evolves. Despite this fact, some authorities claim that early assessment will yield data unusable for patient management and suggest that formal testing should be withheld until stability is achieved. Holland (1983), for example, states that testing at all in the early stages of recovery is a waste of time, and says time would be better used by being "warm" and "using the special skills and tools of the speech pathologist's trade."

There is danger in such a philosophy. No one, in any medical specialty, would or should abandon diagnosis for chitchat and anecdote, regardless of severity or duration or illness. To do so because the patient will change demeans the clinician's skills. Aphasia is dynamic, and so is hemiplegia. Appropriate treatment for both is dynamic as well. Treatment should be responsive to the needs of the patient at any particular time. To withhold treatment because these deficits are not stable is to deny the patient access to the conditions that will improve his or her ability to benefit from treatment; very probably it will also be impossible to recover that lost time, because funding sources are unlikely to support treatment beyond one year. Withholding treatment will also nurture maladaptive and inappropriate behaviors that may require extensive treatment to undo once the patient is stable.

The author advocates early testing because failing to test is a disservice to the patient. Clinicians should not succumb to the siren of subjectivity until the evidence persuades them that they should not resist it. Clinicians do not treat according to the test or to the aphasia. They test early and regularly because their data contribute to the medical management of patients. They test to expose both strengths and weaknesses and to reveal those areas and modes most likely to be improved. When deficits resolve, they change their focus.

Porch (1981) says that the ideal treatment candidate is one whose medical condition is stable, who has a predicted overall percentile significantly above his or her present overall score, and who exhibits variation on item scores within subtests in at least some modalities.

Generally, patients who have suffered a cerebrovascular accident (CVA) are considered medically and neurologically stable by approximately 1 month post onset. Four to 6 weeks is generally considered the end of the period of rapid, spontaneous recovery and the beginning of neurologic and physiologic stability (deBleser and Poeck, 1984, among others). As has been seen, stability is a relative term. Generally, it means that the patient is no longer in acute distress or that his or her condition is no longer critical. It does not mean that the patient will not continue to improve, that his or her condition has plateaued, or that physiological recovery has ended. Physiological recovery, as is well known, seems to continue in many cases for years. Patients untreated for speech and language problems or for hemiplegia return to clinic years later, walking better and talking better. The healing effects of time are often extolled, but not frequently enough in the globally aphasic patient.

As has been noted, there is some evidence to suggest that globally aphasic patients recover differently from other aphasic patients. The typical recovery curve for a single, left hemisphere CVA resulting in aphasia accelerates rapidly in the first month, to approximately 60 to 70 percent of the total recovery. After that time the curve begins to plateau, achieving near stability (at least by our gross measures) at around 1 year post onset. The recovery curve for globally aphasic patients is relatively flat initially, however, and the majority of their recovery may occur after 6 months have elapsed.

Sarno and Levita (1979) compared the response to treatment of 14 globally aphasic patients, 8 fluent aphasic patients, and 12 nonfluent aphasic patients. All 34 patients improved during the 1 year course of treatment. The most striking finding was that, although the globally aphasic patients never reached the levels of the other patients, their greatest percentage of recovery occurred in the period from 6 months to 1 year post onset. This advantage held whether comparing their second 6 months to their first 6 months, or comparing those same periods of recovery to those of the other two groups.

Two additional results from this study are noteworthy. First, none of their globally aphasic patients evolved into a distinctive subtype. Second, globally aphasic patients showed "substantial" recovery during the first year post onset.

Sarno and Levita's results may be related, although they do not so state, to an acceleration of physiological recovery during the second 6 months. There are no empirical data to support this, but it is a reasonable hypothesis to be tested. One possibility, alluded to earlier in this book, is that diaschisis and diminished blood flow may inhibit recovery of speech and language, sometimes for a considerable period of time. It is conceivable that treatment will not yield optimal results until cortical homeostasis is resumed. Conversely, it may be that the first 6 months of treatment is a *necessary* precursor to the improvements made later, and individual variability cannot be discounted. "Waiting for a favorable tide" is a practical approach to surfing and perhaps to treatment, but it is probably best judged individually and not on group data.

Because patients differ in so many ways eventual recovery levels of the patient whose condition is not stable because his or her stroke is still evolving, or whose cardiovascular system continues to release emboli, is difficult to predict. Frequently, the effects of CVA yield a picture of confusion, lethargy, unresponsiveness, listlessness, lassitude, indifference, and sometimes resistance in the early stages of recovery. These behaviors are probably not typical of the patients' premorbid temperament (although they may be extensions of it), and to base a prognosis on behaviors affected by them is premature. Stability should be judged on an individual basis. The noncompliant patient is not necessarily a poor candidate for treatment.

## COMPREHENSIVE MEASURES OF COMMUNICATIVE ABILITY

### Porch Index of Communicative Ability

One of the more popular and enduring diagnostic tests for aphasia is the *Porch Index of Communicative Ability* (PICA) (Porch, 1967). This test samples performance across five communicative modalities (gesturing, writing, speaking, reading, and listening) to ten homogeneous objects. Responses are scored with a 16 point, multidimensional, binary choice scoring system (Table 3–1). Scores are averaged for each of 18 subtests, and modality scores (pantomime, speaking, auditory comprehension, reading, writing, and copying) are obtained by averaging the appropriate scores. The overall score is a mean score derived from all 180 scores, and from that score a percentile can be determined that is based on performance of 375 aphasic adults, Porch's normative sample.

### Boston Diagnostic Aphasia Examination

The *Boston Diagnostic Aphasia Examination* (BDAE) (Goodglass and Kaplan, 1983) is another popular test for determining overall communicative ability. The test was designed to meet three general aims: (1) diag-

**Table 3–1.    The PICA Categories for Scoring Responses**

| Score | Category | Dimensional Characteristics |
|-------|----------|------------------------------|
| 16 | Complex | Accurate, responsive, complex, prompt, efficient |
| 15 | Complete | Accurate, responsive, complete, prompt, efficient |
| 14 | Distorted | Accurate, responsive, complete or complex, prompt, distorted |
| 13 | Complete-Delayed | Accurate, responsive, complete or complex, delayed |
| 12 | Incomplete | Accurate, responsive, incomplete, prompt |
| 11 | Incomplete-Delayed | Accurate, responsive, incomplete, delayed |
| 10 | Corrected | Accurate, self-corrected |
| 9 | Repeated | Accurate, after instructions are repeated |
| 8 | Cued | Accurate, after cue is given |
| 7 | Related | Inaccurate, almost accurate |
| 6 | Error | Inaccurate attempt at the task item |
| 5 | Intelligible | Comprehensible but not an attempt at the task item |
| 4 | Unintelligible | Incomprehensible but differentiated |
| 3 | Minimal | Incomprehensible and undifferentiated |
| 2 | Attention | No response, but patient attends to the tester |
| 1 | No Response | No response, no awareness of task |

nosis of presence and type of aphasic syndrome, leading to inferences concerning cerebral localization; (2) measurement of the level of performance over a wide range, for both initial determination and detection of change over time; (3) comprehensive assessment of the assets and liabilities of the patient in all areas as a guide to therapy. An earlier version of the test (Goodglass and Kaplan, 1972) ignored global aphasia. The new version of the test includes global aphasia and provides a very useful addition, percentiles in place of z-scores.

The test includes sections for the assessment of conversational and expository speech, auditory comprehension, oral expression, understanding written language, and writing. Scoring is primarily plus-minus, although speech characteristics (melodic line, phrase length, articulatory agility, grammatical form, paraphasia, and word finding) are rated on a 7 point, equal-appearing interval scale. One appealing feature of the test is its comprehensiveness. In addition to the assessment of communicative skills, the authors provide tests for disconnection syndromes, a "parietal lobe" battery, and tests for nonverbal apraxia. Duffy (1979), who praised the test (but with a few misgivings), wrote

Those clinicians who are more interested in aphasia as a multidimensional disorder and whose purpose for testing is to evaluate severity of communi-

cative impairment, make prognostic statements, and plan treatment programs, may find other tests . . . better suited to their needs. (p. 201)

Those tests include the PICA, the *Minnesota Test for Differential Diagnosis of Aphasia (MTDDA)* (Schuell, 1965), or the *Western Aphasia
Battery* (Kertesz, 1982).

## The Western Aphasia Battery

The *Western Aphasia Battery* (WAB) is another comprehensive test for
aphasia. An earlier, unpublished version has evolved into a comprehensive, valid, and reliable measure for aphasia severity. It is designed to
evaluate content, fluency, auditory comprehension, repetition, naming,
reading, writing, and calculation, and assesses nonverbal skills, including drawing, block design, and praxis. The nonverbal tests, which
include the RCPM, are optional. Their inclusion provides a more complete picture of deficits than many tests permit.

Scoring is generally plus-minus, but with some interesting and useful variations. Scoring of spontaneous speech, for example, reflects two
fundamental dimensions, information content and fluency, in response
to six general questions and a picture description. Scores for each dimension range from 0 to 10, for a maximum combined score of 20. Scores of
0 are given for no information or for no words or short, meaningless
utterances. Scores of 10 reflect correct responses to all six items, with
sentences of normal length and complexity referring to most of the items
and activities, and a reasonably complete description of the picture, ren-
dered in sentences of normal length and complexity, without definite
slowing, halting, or articulatory difficulties and no paraphasias.

Information content generally interacts with fluency, grammatical
completeness, and paraphasias, but there is not necessarily a correspondence between ratings on either dimension. Use of both dimensions cap-
tures both the richness and paucity of expression, but the total score
does not reveal that richness.

Subscores are summed for spontaneous speech, comprehension,
repetition, and naming, and the subscore totals are divided to derive an
aphasia quotient (AQ). A cortical quotient (CQ) can be derived from
reading and writing, praxis, and construction scores.

Normal subjects achieve AQs of 100 to 93.8. The lower score was
selected by the author as an arbitrary boundary for normal performance. Globally aphasic patients, on the other hand, produce scores in
each of the categories composing the oral language section (fluency,
comprehension, repetition, and naming), which range from 0 to 6. Best
performance by globally aphasic patients would not yield an AQ of

greater than 37.6 and would range downward to 0 in the most severe cases.

Because it is comprehensive, relatively easy to score and administer, and provides an adequate data base for most aphasic subtypes, particularly for globally aphasic patients, the WAB is an appealing alternative to other, traditional tests for aphasia.

The tests discussed hitherto are said to be comprehensive in that they sample a variety of communicative behaviors across traditional communicative modalities. One, the PICA, assesses communicative ability on homogeneous items of equal difficulty across 18 subtests of decreasing difficulty and relies on a multidimensional scoring system to reveal subtle differences in performance. Both the WAB and the BDAE assess communicative ability on a variety of relatively heterogeneous language tasks.

Few tests have sufficient breadth to provide thorough assessment of aphasia and related disorders. Many clinicians prefer to administer multiple tests or only portions of a number of tests. This shotgun approach is useful for experienced clinicians, but there are some disadvantages. First, few clinicians have an adequate data base for comparisons of performance. Second, the units selected may, because they are taken from a unified test, compromise the intent and results of the test. Because standardization is violated, results become less meaningful.

Isolated "windows" or relatively intact communicative skills are not always revealed when the assessment is confined to one standard assessment tool. Although the efficiency of formal, standardized testing permits better use of the clinician's and patient's time, thorough assessment requires a battery of tests.

## TESTS FOR APRAXIA

Tests for apraxia of speech yield little valuable information in global aphasia. For that reason they are not discussed in this section. If there is a sufficient variety and spontaneity of speech production to warrant this test, chances are good that the patient is not globally aphasic or will not be for long.

The prevalence of limb apraxia in global aphasia is not a hollow issue. Its presence may be difficult to detect, but when limb apraxia is present it may have a significant effect on some avenues of therapeutic intervention. A typical test for oral, nonverbal apraxia and limb apraxia is shown in Table 3–2.

Many of these commands, presented auditorially, will elicit appropriate responses if the apraxia is mild. In the most severe forms of global

## Table 3–2. Tests for Oral and Limb Apraxia

PATIENT _____ DATE _____ EXAMINER _____

Give each item twice on command and once on imitation regardless of the patient's adequacy. Directions for the first presentation are: "I'm going to ask you to do some things with your tongue and mouth. Listen carefully and do exactly what I ask you to do. " For the second: "All right, let's try it again. " For the third: "Okay, now watch me carefully and do exactly what I do. "

| Score each response: | Trial 1 | Repeat | Cue |
|---|---|---|---|
| 1.  Open your mouth. | _____ | _____ | _____ |
| 2.  Stick out your tongue. | _____ | _____ | _____ |
| 3.  Show me how you blow. | _____ | _____ | _____ |
| 4.  Show me your teeth. | _____ | _____ | _____ |
| 5.  Pucker up your lips. | _____ | _____ | _____ |
| 6.  Puff out your cheeks. | _____ | _____ | _____ |
| 7.  Bite your lower lip. | _____ | _____ | _____ |
| 8.  Show me how you whistle. | _____ | _____ | _____ |
| 9.  Lick your lips all the way around. | _____ | _____ | _____ |
| 10.  Clear your throat. | _____ | _____ | _____ |
| 1.  Show me how you salute. | _____ | _____ | _____ |
| 2.  Make the letter "o" with your fingers. | _____ | _____ | _____ |
| 3.  Make a fist. | _____ | _____ | _____ |
| 4.  Shake your finger at me. | _____ | _____ | _____ |
| 5.  Show me how you play a piano. | _____ | _____ | _____ |
| 6.  Show me how to play an accordion. | _____ | _____ | _____ |
| 7.  Wave good-bye. | _____ | _____ | _____ |
| 8.  Show me how you scratch. | _____ | _____ | _____ |
| 9.  Show me how to hammer. | _____ | _____ | _____ |
| 10.  Make the sign for victory. | _____ | _____ | _____ |

Mayo Clinic Procedures for Language Evaluation, unpublished.

aphasia, most commands will not be understood or, if the apraxia is severe as well, will not be carried out initially. The severity of the comprehension deficit prevents accurate assessment of praxis. More useful information is provided by assessment in three conditions: to command, to repetition of that command, and to imitation. In milder forms of aphasia, when apraxia is present the apraxia is revealed in differential performance between imitation and command. In more severe forms, responses may be elicited only through imitation, and assessment of apraxia is made through quality of response to each task.

The oral, nonverbal apraxia and limb apraxia battery is much more useful when responses are scored in some multidimensional manner. Many scoring systems exist and none are problem-free. The scoring system shown in Table 3-3 is relatively responsive to clinical requirements, but clinicians may prefer the system shown in Table 3-4.

## TESTING AUDITORY COMPREHENSION

Only three popular tests for aphasia assess comprehension of "yes" and "no": The BDAE, the WAB, and the MTDDA, despite the crucial importance of that response to communication. The BDAE assesses yes-no ability through a series of complex sentences and corresponding sentences that yield the opposite answer—for example, "Will a cork sink in water?" and "Will a stone sink in water?"—and four questions following the oral reading of four informational paragraphs.

The MTDDA questions assess that ability through questions about previously learned material (e.g., "Do we get milk from cows?"). The WAB asks twenty yes-no questions, ten requiring "no" for a response and ten requiring "yes," (for example, "Are you in a hotel?" and "Is your name _____?").

Clinician-constructed yes-no assessments are similar in design and intent: they ask an equal number of yes-no questions and often pair opposites, either one immediately following the other or later in the test.

Gray, Hoyt, Mogil, and Lefkowitz (1977) examined the performance of aphasic patients on the yes-no section of the BDAE, WAB, and MTDDA. They made the following observations:

1.  Significantly more errors were made to BDAE (informational questions) than to WAB or MTDDA.
2.  Patients were more likely to answer "yes" when questions became difficult.
3.  Significantly fewer errors occurred on personal than on environmental questions, and the most errors occurred on informational questions.
4.  The WAB, which is sensitive to a broad spectrum of semantic questions, is more appropriate for severely impaired patients than BDAE or MTDDA.

Responses to yes-no questions became less predictable as task complexity and demands increased. Performance was better on tasks requiring responses related to self (whole body commands, family names, and so forth).

## Table 3–3.  Scoring for Tests of Oral and Limb Apraxia

| | |
|---|---|
| 11 | Correct without delay. |
| 10 | Correct after delay during which no oral movement is observed, except for that accompaning verbalizing the instructions. |
| 9 | Self-corrected response. Patient performs discrete gesture(s) and then corrects. |
| 8 | Partial response. Patient response could be identified by the intact elements but a part of a gesture is missing or mildly altered. |
| 7 | Augmented response. Something is added to an identifiable performance of the response. Not to be assigned if the result of augmentation is another discrete gesture present in the battery. |
| 6 | Patient engages in groping trial and error behavior before settling on the correct response. |
| 5 | Patient makes a discrete incorrect gesture. |
| 4 | Groping trial and error behavior never results in correct response but differs from other trial and error efforts. |
| 3 | Undifferentiated groping. |
| 2 | Minimal. Attention and minimal movement or recognition. |
| 1 | No response. |

*Add to the above numbers:*

| | |
|---|---|
| P | if response has obvious perseverative elements |
| S | if response is accompanied by or is solely speech noise |
| D | if response is slowed or disturbed by dysarthria |

Mayo Clinic Procedures for Language Evaluation, unpublished.

In theory, aphasia severity should predict differential performance across this spectrum of difficulty. The yes-no questions that follow parallel, at least in theory, such a hierarchy of difficulty. The questions should be asked at a predetermined comfortable level of loudness for the patient, allowing ample time to respond (5 to 30 seconds) and approximately 5 seconds between questions. Verbal or gestural responses should be recorded as correct. It is a good idea, by the way, to ask only questions to which you know the answer. Sample questions are shown in Table 3-5.

Responses to these questions should allow the clinician to determine the integrity of this response and, more importantly, to convey that information to staff and family.

Gray and colleagues (1977) reported that patients were more likely to respond "yes" than "no." Acquiescence appears to be easier than negation, for globally aphasic patients as well as other people. Persistent affirmation will, of course, result in a score of 15 of 30 correct, or chance performance. If the patient appears to be guessing, the clinician should restate and ask the 15 "no" questions. Chances are the score will plummet below the chance level.

**Table 3–4.  Alternative Scoring for Tests of Oral and Limb Apraxia**

| | |
|---|---|
| 8 | Accurate, immediate, on command |
| 7 | Accurate, after trial and error, searching movements, on command |
| 6 | Crude, defective in amplitude, accuracy, or speed, on command |
| 5 | Partial, important part missing, on command |
| 4 | Same as 8, after demonstration |
| 3 | Same as 7, after demonstration |
| 2 | Same as 6, after demonstration |
| 1 | Same as 5, after demonstration |
| OP | Perseverative |
| OI | Irrelevant; some other oral performance, including speech |
| ON | Nil, no oral performance |

Mayo Clinic Procedures for Language Evaluation, unpublished.

More traditional tests of auditory comprehension include the *Token Test* (DeRenzi and Vignolo, 1962) and the *Revised Token Test* (McNeil and Prescott, 1978). These tests are not entirely inappropriate for the globally aphasic patient, but the inability of global patients to perform all but a few of the tasks makes their results unrevealing.

## TESTING READING COMPREHENSION

The *Reading Comprehension Battery for Aphasia* (LaPointe and Horner, 1979) is probably the most appropriate reading test for severe aphasia. It is relatively short (ten subtests of ten items each), and assesses single-word comprehension relative to visual, auditory, and semantic confusions as well as a range of reading comprehension skills from functional sentences through paragraphs and more difficult morphosyntactic reading.

At this time the normative base is inadequate for comparisons to samples other than those for normal adults. Performance for globally aphasic patients can be expected to fall dramatically after the reading recognition subtests to nearly a chance level.

## ASSESSMENT OF WRITING

The assessment of writing has been addressed in a structured format by only a few authors. As do some other tests, the PICA, BDAE, and WAB assess writing in progressively more difficult tasks and rate mechanics and context according to predetermined criteria. No tests designed solely

**Table 3–5.  Questions Eliciting "Yes" and "No" Responses**

Personal                                                                                                    Score

1.  Is your name (correct name)?

2.  Is your name (incorrect name)?

3.  Do you live in (incorrect name)?

4.  Do you live in (correct name)?

5.  Are you a doctor?

6.  Are you (appropriate occupation or retired)?

7.  Are you wearing a _____ ? (answer should be no)

8.  Are you wearing a _____ ? (answer should be yes)

9.  Do you have _____ hair? (yes)

10.  Do you have _____ hair? (no)

*Immediate Environment*

1.  Are you in the hospital?

2.  Are you in a movie?

3.  Is the light on?

4.  Is the light off?

5.  Do you live in _____ ? (yes)

6.  Are you in _____ ? (no)

7.  Is there a _____ in this room? (no)

8.  Is there a _____ in this room? (yes)

9.  Is the door closed? (yes)

10.  Is the door open? (no)

*Informational*

1.  Does January follow June? (no)

2.  Does spring come before fall? (yes)

3.  Is a window made of glass? (yes)

4.  Do you light a cigarette with a chair? (no)

5.  Is five more than two? (yes)

6.  Do people sleep on a table? (no)

7.  Does milk come from a cow? (yes)

8.  Does Coke come from a cow? (no)

9.  Do you catch fish with a bus? (no)

10.  Do you tell time with a watch? (yes)          Mean Score:

for the assessment of writing in aphasia exist. Clinical assessment of writing is usually done in a top to bottom fashion, depending on the results obtained in formal testing. The patient is asked to write his (or her) name and address. If the patient is unable to write or writes unintelligibly, have him copy his name. If he is unable to copy his name, try having him copy single letters or simple geometric shapes until you are able to form an impression based on the patient's efforts.

Raven's *Coloured Progressive Matrices* (Raven, 1962) is a widely used test of nonverbal, visual problem-solving ability in aphasia and related disorders. Theoretically, the abilities assessed by this measure are relatively well-preserved in aphasia. Poorer performance suggests cognitive deficits that are unrelated to the aphasia.

In general, the correlation of this measure with language measures is small and does not reach significance. In patients with more severe handicaps, however, the relationship is much more substantial and may be a particularly powerful prognostic indicator.

## FUNCTIONAL COMMUNICATION ASSESSMENT

Questionnaires can be an excellent source of information about the globally aphasic patient. One such questionnaire is an adaptation of the *Functional Communication Profile* (Sarno, 1969) (see Appendix A) and is unpublished (modified by Collins, 1980). A similar measure, also an adaptation of the FCP, was employed by Wertz and colleagues (1981). Called the *Rating of Functional Performance,* it is an amalgamation of several earlier tests. Behaviors are rated on a 5 point scale ranging from "1" (cannot do what is asked in the question) to "5" (no difficulty in doing what is asked in the question and ability to do it as well as people who have not had a stroke). The scale is simplified, and the number of categories is reduced because it was designed to be administered by a spouse, friend, or caregiver. Clinicians who use the scale may want to use another scoring system.

The test assesses strengths and weaknesses in five modalities (recognition or understanding; responding; reading; speaking; writing) in addition to an "other" category for behaviors that were unclassifiable by traditional modalities, such as "Can he keep track of time?" and "Can he use money appropriately?" It appears to be useful not only as a baseline and diagnostic measure but also as a means of focusing treatment on functional, needed skills and as a measure of progress.

This scale is designed to be completed by a person familiar with the patient, but it may be filled out in an interview format. There are five sections to the form, which covers understanding, reading, speaking, writing, and an "other" category. Abilities are rated on a scale of 1 to 5. This scale ranges from "never," "poor" (usually cannot do what is asked but has done it infrequently since the stroke); "fair" (can do what is asked about half the time); "good" (can do what is asked most of the time); to "normal" (can perform the task as well as people who have not had a stroke).

The questions are arranged in a hierarchy from simple to difficult. They may be particularly well-suited to the severely or globally aphasic patient because they sample a range of behaviors not sampled in traditional tests. The clinician may rate the behaviors in lieu of a rater close to the patient, or both the clinician and the other rater may rate the behaviors. The clinicians should interpret the results cautiously. There is some evidence to suggest that there is relatively poor agreement between clinicians' ratings of communicative behaviors and ratings made by significant others (Wertz et al., 1981). The reasons for this are unclear, but it may be that, if these people are not more astute observers, they are at least more practiced observers of that particular patient. It may also be that they are less objective than clinicians and more willing to attribute certain abilities to a patient than clinicians are. They may also be less careful in controlling for artifacts. Nevertheless, a measure such as this is an important adjunct to diagnostic procedures.

Another potentially useful measure is the *Rating of Patient's Independence* (ROPI) (Porch and Collins, 1974). This scale rates communicative, nonverbal, and other, noncommunicative abilities on a 15 point, multidimensional, binary-choice rating scale. The scoring system is reliable, but its validity has not been examined.

Perhaps the most useful feature is the rating scale, which incorporates four dimensions: independence, versatility, consistency, and ability. The major criterion for quality of performance is independence. Ratings of 8 (independent in some aspects of the task, performs those aspects of the task inconsistently [50 to 90 percent of the time] with reduced ability) to 15 (independent in all aspects of the task, performs the task consistently with normal [premorbid] ability) generally reflect independent functioning, whereas scores of 7 and below reflect diminishing ability to perform tasks and performance always requiring supervision.

## Formal Assessment of Functional Communication

The *Functional Communication Profile* (FCP) (Sarno, 1969) is a test designed to assess the language performance of aphasic patients in informal settings. It differs from other, more traditional tests in that it measures "functional performance. . .the unforced, voluntary, and habitual utterances which characterize normal spoken language" (p. 1). Although the test is "nontask oriented," 45 specific communication behaviors, rated on a 9 point scale during a conversation between a speech pathologist and a patient, are divided into five categories: movement, speaking, understanding, reading, and a miscellaneous category that includes writing and calculation. The examiner sums the ratings and then uses a conversion chart to derive a weighted score and an overall percentage indicating the patient's effectiveness in everyday communication. "Normal" performance on the scale refers to the clinician's judgment of the patient's premorbid abilities, derived from the information about age, educational level, and employment. The test makes allowances for compensatory behaviors, such as gesturing when speech is called for. Other nonlinguistic factors, such as speed, accuracy, and consistency of performance, are considered in arriving at ratings. The test takes little time to administer (10 to 20 minutes) and is valid and reliable.

Holland (1977) also recognized the distinction between measurable, verbal behaviors and what has been called communicative competence. Communicative competence refers to "knowledge of the rules of social discourse in a given language; it includes things like knowing who speaks to whom, what is rude and what is polite, and when to speak and when to be silent," among other things. Her belief, and that of most clinicians, is that communicative competence is not lost in aphasia, even when the deficits are global. Holland observed that "aphasics probably communicate better than they talk," and she has devised a test in response to a void in aphasia assessment and treatment, the adequacy of communication in simulated daily life activities.

Holland's test (1980), *Communicative Abilities in Daily Living* (CADL), is composed of 68 items, can be administered in 35 to 40 minutes, is reliable, and has a high concurrent validity with other, more traditional tests of aphasia. It may be a particularly appropriate adjunct for appraising the abilities of the globally aphasic patient. Most tests are modality-bound and task-specific, but this test makes allowances for compensatory behaviors—for example, gesturing when a spoken message is called for. The salient communicative act to be scored is "getting the message across," and verbal and nonverbal responses have equal potential for being scored in the same manner.

The CADL employs a 3 point scoring system (0, 1, and 2). A score of 0 is given for a "wrong" response, a score of 1 for an "adequate" response, and a score of 2 for a "correct" response. If the message the patient sends is clearly understood by the tester, the response is considered to be correct. For example, item 35 requires the patient to read an automobile fuel gauge setting on empty, showing the car to be out of gas. Examples of responses rating 2 points include the following: "It's empty gas"; "Car is out of gas"; "It depends on whether the engine is running; if so, it's almost out of gas, or the gas gauge is broken or, if the engine isn't running, it doesn't mean anything at all"; or pointing to the gas gauge and shaking the head "no." An "adequate" response (1 point) to the same item would include pointing to the gauge, but not in any elaborating way or indicating the relationship between it and the idea of emptiness.

The test is designed to provide different information about an aphasic patient than other traditional tests and is intended to supplement, rather than substitute for, other measures. Traditional measures are designed to minimize the contextual cues people frequently use in daily living. The CADL attempts to incorporate both more natural language activities and a more natural style in an effort to approximate normal communication. Other nonlinguistic variables, such as speed, accuracy, and consistency of performance, are considered in arriving at ratings.

The test has a demonstrably high correlation with other "formal" tests of communicative ability (Holland, 1980). Holland found that the CADL correlated highly with two of the more traditional tests for aphasia: .93 for the PICA and .84 for the BDAE. Some authors, however, have reported a lack of agreement between task-oriented test and functional ratings. Sarno and Levita (1979), for example, were "impressed with the lack of correspondence between task-oriented performance and functional ratings" (p. 668). The discrepancy in these findings is difficult to explain, but it may be related to the measures used.

The high correlations obtained by Holland may be reassuring to those who believe that formal measures such as the PICA have high content validity as well as high predictive validity—that is, to other situations and other communicative environments. Statistical significance, however, can be misleading or inappropriate when applied to individual patients or to other settings, and it does not tell, for example, what critical information is lost, or unexplained, in that correlation. It may be that the unexplained variance (somewhere between 7 and 16 percent) reflects that much error in the correlations, but it does not mean that information captured by one test is not captured by the other. What information is not captured, and by which test(s), and whether the particular information is critical are questions that are as yet unanswered. The most conservative approach is probably a compromise between sampling and thorough testing. If one test does not allow a patient to display a more complete repertoire of the things he or she can do, the clinician should provide a forum for those skills through supplemental tests.

Because most aphasia tests attempt to capture the abilities of mildly to moderately affected patients, crucial information about residual nonverbal communication skills in severe aphasia is not revealed. "This is especially true when referring to global aphasia where the difference between *total absence* of word production and the ability to use even a few words in everyday life can make a substantial difference in the individual's relationship to the real world" (Sarno and Levita, p. 668).

Edelman (1984), among others, recognized the need for more discriminating tests for global aphasia, particularly with respect to the measurement of comprehension. She says there are no tests that are sensitive to the skills that remain intact in global aphasia. The framework Edelman suggests calls for the systematic evaluation of understanding both in and out of context and in the absence and presence of variables that may be facilitative. Her test has not been standardized, is unpublished, and is still in the process of development. Nevertheless, it promises to contribute significantly to our understanding of global aphasia and to direct our treatment to enhance those skills. An outline of the test format, with sample questions, follows:

I.   Screening Procedures
    A.   Responds to greeting or lateralizes to sound
    B.   Establishes or maintains eye contact

II.  Commands
    A.   Relating to self
        1.   Whole body commands
            a.   Look at me
            b.   Lean forward
        2.   Limb movements
            a.   Show me your arm
            b.   Squeeze my hand
        3.   Orofacial movements
            a.   Stick out your tongue
            b.   Show me how you smile
    B.   Relating to objects in the environment
        1.   Recognition
            a.   In meaningful context
               example: raises leg in physical therapy when asked
            b.   Acontextually
               example: raises leg in speech when asked

        2.   Manipulation
            a.   In meaningful context
               example: uses a spoon correctly at lunch
            b.   Acontextually
               example: uses a spoon correctly in speech when asked
    C.   Questions
        1.   Relating to self: high affective content
            a.   Is your name _____ ?
            b.   Is your wife's (husband's) name _____ ?

2.   Relating to environment: low affective content
   a.   Is the light on?
   b.   Is the chair green?

To enhance the sensitivity of the test, Edelman (1984) uses a hierarchy of cues. In this hierarchy, the examiner first states the command or question, but may repeat it if necessary and at a slowed rate. If the patient fails to respond correctly at those levels, the utterance may be expanded. If the first three attempts fail, a gesture may accompany the question or command. To expand the question "Are you married?" the clinician might ask "Are you married? Do you have a wife?" To enhance a question, the examiner might repeat the question and gesture to a ring finger.

To provide even more sensitivity, Edelman (1984) has incorporated a modified PICA scoring system. This 10 point system is multidimensional, reflecting accuracy, completeness, promptness, and responsiveness. The scoring system is as follows:

10   Accurate, complete, prompt
9    Accurate, complete, but slowed or delayed
8    Accurate after self-correction of error
7    Accurate after repetition of instruction
6    Accurate after verbal expansion of instruction
5    Accurate after gestural cue
4    Inaccurate but related to correct response
3    Inaccurate
2    Attention to test item but no response
1    No response—no apparent awareness of test items

Houghton, Pettit, and Towey (1982) have developed a test called the *Communicative Competence Evaluation Instrument* (CCEI), which consists of 20 (10 expressive and 10 receptive) communicative competence behaviors. This test combines elements of the FCP, *Components of Communicative Competence Scale* (CCCS) (Malone, 1978), and the *Interaction Process Analysis System* (IPA) (Bales, 1970). Responses to both verbal and nonverbal spoken and gestured directions can be rated, and a patient is allowed credit for either verbal or nonverbal expression.

Five minute videotaped samples of each patient's performance are made before and after treatment, and the behaviors are rated on a 6 point scale. The ratings correspond to judgments of "behaviors not observed" (1) through "fair" (3) to "excellent" (6). This brief test is reliable and has at least face validity, but concurrent validity has not been examined.

## In Vivo Observations

One final, informal measurement should be discussed: observation in vivo. Because the data are expensive to gather and the observations frequently intrusive, this method is probably not practiced often.

Holland (1982) is probably the foremost proponent of observation of aphasic patients at work and at play. She has proposed a system for describing communicative behaviors in varied situations. Holland observed the communicative behaviors of 40 aphasic patients for approximately 2 hours, and rated their communication, or attempts at communication, as successes (appropriate) or failures (inappropriate). The categories she used for these ratings follow:

*Verbal Output*
  Form:  Verbal lubricant, social convention
         Asks questions, makes requests
         Answers questions or responds to requests
         Volunteers information
  Style:  Agrees or disagrees
         Teases, uses humor or sarcasm
         Metaphor
  Conversational dominance:   Interrupts or changes topics
  Correctional strategies:   Corrects, clarifies, requests
  Metalinguistics:   Comments on own speaking
                     Responds to phonemic cues

*Nonverbal Output*
  Spatial indicators
  Direct verbal referrant
  Gestures to maintain conversation
  Humor
  Affect or state

*Read, Write, Mathematical Ability, and Similar Skills*
  Responds to written material
  Writes
  Responds to numbers

*Other*
  Talks on phone
  Talks to pets
  Talks to self
  Responds to household sounds
  Sings
  Speaks in foreign languages

Although none of Holland's subjects (1982) were classified as having global aphasia (using the 1972 version of the BDAE), the range of scores was as low as 8.13 on the PICA. Presumably, at least one of her "mixed" subjects had global aphasia.

By tallying frequency of both failed and successful communicative acts, Holland found that there were significantly more successes than failures, perhaps indicating that most patients attempt to communicate when they think they can, and in their chosen compensated manner.

This system for identifying behaviors is particularly useful in the structure it provides for thinking about communication in patients who are primarily nonverbal, but who can communicate.

## SUMMARY

The assessment measures discussed in this chapter are representative of those used in many clinics in the United States and in some other countries (for example, the U.K. and Canada) as well. Some tests were slighted or went unnoticed. This slighting was deliberate but not judgmental. There are other tests that clinicians will be more comfortable with and in their hands are just as powerful. This review in this chapter is biased in two ways: to reflect the author's philosophy that assessment should be a compromise among brevity, thoroughness, and attention to behaviors that can be measured adequately and efficiently as they change; and his experience with measures that highlight salient variables.

In Chapter 4, prediction of recovery is discussed. In large part the prognoses given there are based on the measures discussed in this chapter. Where and when questions or doubts persist, intuition and subjectivity are called on. But because the author believes that patient management is too important to leave to caprice and serendipity, an attempt has been made to provide tentative structure to that informality to help guide clinicians to valid answers to their hypotheses.

A summary of assessment measures in common clinical use is shown in Table 3-6. Administering all the listed tests is unnecessary and forbiddingly tiring for clinician and patient alike. Generally, choosing one of the measures of general communicative ability and using selected tests, including measures of functional communication, for more fine-tuned testing in each modality, is adequate.

**Table 3–6.  Assessing Global Aphasia: Suggested Formal and Informal Measures**

Informal Assessment
    Family or caregiver interview
    Medical record review
    Patient interview
    Consultation with other rehabilitation services

Formal Assessment: Standardized Tests
    *Porch Index of Communicative Ability*
    *Western Aphasia Battery*
    *Boston Diagnostic Aphasia Examination*

Reading
    *Reading Comprehension Battery for Aphasia*

Auditory Comprehension
    *Token Test*
    *Revised Token Test*

Naming
    *Boston Naming Test*

Speech
    *Standard Speech Sample*

Other
    *Coloured Progressive Matrices*

Nonstandardized Assessment
    General
        *Mayo Clinic Procedures for Language Evaluation*

Reading
    Clinician constructed tests of single-word and sentence material of patient-salient
    materials
    a.  matching
    b.  word recognition with one or more foils
    Body-part and nonbody-part instructions

Auditory Comprehension
    Yes-no questions
    Body commands
    Nonbody commands

Speech
    Serial responses
    a.  count to 20
    b.  days of the week
    c.  months of the year
    Sentence completion
    Repetition
        a.  single words
        b.  sentences
        c.  patient-salient material

Writing
    Copying letters
    Copying single words

Writing name and address
Copying name and address
Writing single letters to dictation
Copying single letters
Copying simple geometric shapes
Writing single words to dictation
Copying of the same words

Apraxia
Assessment of oral, nonverbal apraxia
Assessment of limb apraxia
Testing with objects-gesture

Functional Communication
*Functional Communication Profile*
*Communicative Abilities in Daily Living*

Questionnaires
*Functional Rating Scale*
*Rating of Functional Performance*
*Rating of Patient's Independence*
*Communicative Competence Evaluation Instrument*

# Chapter 4

# Predicting Recovery

Few of the clinicians' skills are as important or as difficult to learn as the prediction of eventual recovery. Making accurate predictions requires a synthesis of experience and data, tempered with the knowledge that clinicians are limited in their powers of observation. Despite a clinical acumen, however, inevitably some patients will escape the clinicians' confidence intervals. Because the predictions clinicians make will affect the lives of both patients and families, we have sufficient reason to be humble and cautious when making them.

Attempting to predict eventual recovery levels may appear to be simply a clinical game that pits the clinician's skills against the patient's response to treatment and physiological recovery of cortical mechanisms. But there are more significant reasons to aim for early and accurate prediction, however. Prediction of recovery permits more effective use of clinical time and, more important, helps the patient and family make crucial and timely decisions about social and occupational planning. Also, in an increasingly restrictive atmosphere for funding of rehabilitation, clinicians are expected to justify treatment decisions.

A stroke is a traumatic event for both patient and family. It alters family dynamics, and traditionally independent people become dependent. Their return to work is a rare occurrence, even in mild aphasia (McAleese, Collins, Rosenbek, and Hengst, 1984) and virtually impossible in global aphasia. Often faced with an early retirement, aphasic men and women are confronted with too much time, too little to do, and inadequate resources. Hobbies, for those who had them, become impossible, because of the aphasia and its associated deficits. Early and informed clinical decisions, even if they must be amended at a later date, may make the transition easier, and, perhaps, make the spouse's assumption of anticipated burdens less devastating.

There are basically three approaches to predicting change in aphasia: prognostic variable; behavioral profile; and statistical prediction.

## PROGNOSTIC VARIABLE APPROACH

In this approach, the clinician compares a patient's biographical, medical, and behavioral profile against those variables believed to influence change in aphasia. Age, etiologic basis, general health, and recency of onset, for example, are believed to influence eventual recovery levels. Conflicting variables, however, are common and present a prognostic predicament.

## BEHAVIORAL PROFILE APPROACH

This method (Keenan and Brassell, 1974; Schuell, 1965; Porch, 1967, 1983) compares performance on formal measures of communication with a profile of change made by similar patients with similar profiles.

Keenan and Brassell (1974) reviewed the clinical records of 39 aphasic patients and identified and correlated three nonlanguage variables (age, general health, and regularity of employment) with six language variables (listening, talking, reading, writing, motor speech impairment, and speech stimulability) on the *Minnesota Test for Differential Diagnosis of Aphasia* (Schuell, 1965) and found that these variables were highly predictive of eventual recovery. Their article was written in an era of relatively unsophisticated brain imaging techniques; newer techniques are capable of providing another prognostic variable, lesion volume, which may add to the power of prediction.

Several methods that are similar to the behavioral profile approach were developed by Porch and others (Porch, 1967, 1983; Porch and Collins, unpublished data, 1973). Each of these procedures is linked to the *Porch Index of Communicative Ability* (PICA), the individual and mean subtest scores, recovery curves generated by responses of a large number of aphasic patients, and variability of performance within and across subtests.

In the first of these, the patient's overall scores at 1 month post onset are compared to a mean subtest score for the aphasic sample, and the predicted outcome for that patient at 6 months post onset is the mean of the nine highest subtests. An overall score of 7.83, for example, places the patient at the 20th percentile. The corresponding "high" score, 10.41, is that patient's projected performance at 6 months post onset, which corresponds to the 45th percentile.

This method is surprisingly accurate, perhaps because the initial overall score is so highly correlated with scores at 6 months and 1 year post onset. Nevertheless, at least one other variable seems to influence the accuracy of prediction. In an unpublished study, Porch and Collins (unpublished data, 1973) found that, even with relatively imprecise estimates of time spent in treatment, those who received substantial amounts of treatment tended to exceed their predicted scores, while those who received minimal or no treatment tended to fall short of their predicted scores.

For those patients beyond 1 month post onset but not past 6 months post onset, an alternative, the High Overall Prediction (HOAP) slopes, is preferable. In this procedure, a prediction is determined by finding the approximate severity level, at the appropriate time post onset, from the family of recovery curves, and estimating the 6 month recovery point.

Finally, although little empirical evidence is available to support its use, Porch discusses the use of intrasubtest variability, which he also calls Peak Mean Difference (PMD) to both predict potential for change and potential response to treatment. It is a refinement of his notion that, with a few notable exceptions, the patient's best performance points toward a potential level of performance. For example, a patient whose mean performance on a given subtest is 10.9, but who has one or more scores above that (e.g., a 15), is indicating that his competence is superior to his performance. Variability is defined as the difference between the mean score and the highest score. A total variability score is obtained by adding variability scores for all 18 subtests.

Variability is generally greatest in the early stages of a patient's recovery. One advantage of the variability index, however, is that it is not tied to time post onset. High variability scores, regardless of duration of aphasia, suggest at least the potential for recovery. Porch suggests that high PMD scores (400 and above) suggest excellent potential for recovery, and that low PMD scores (below 200) suggest poor capacity for improvement. Examples for the use of these predictions are included later when case histories are presented.

## STATISTICAL PREDICTION

One final prediction method should be mentioned. It has not been fully tested, but appears somewhat feasible. Porch, Collins, Wertz, and Friden (1980) used a stepwise multiple regression procedure that attempts to predict recovery levels at 3, 6, and 12 months post onset from PICA data obtained at 1, 3, and 6 months post onset. Working with data obtained from 144 aphasic patients, Porch and colleagues found that accuracy of prediction increased as the interval from onset decreased, but that all correlations were significant. Gestural, verbal, and graphic modality scores and age were the four predictive variables used. Surprisingly, age was a significant factor in only two of the six equations generated. Gestural scores were the most consistently significant predictors.

The results of this study are potentially significant. The generation of accurate formulae for prediction permits the creation of a prognosis using an individual's own language to predict change rather than making comparisons to group performance. At the present time, the method is more promising than useful. Replication with larger samples of aphasic patients, and the inclusion of additional variables such as treatment frequency, intensity, and type should enhance clinicians' ability to predict.

## VARIABILITY IN TEST AND SUBTEST SCORES

Preeminent among Porch's criteria for prediction of good recovery is significant variation in scores within subtests, or significant variation in modality scores. Porch suggests that the variations in performance may be more important than the overall score because they suggest a competence in communicative abilities that is not revealed in the scores contributing to the depressions in performance. In other words, the ability to perform a task at a particular level, however occasionally, indicates that this "best" performance can be produced more frequently, more consistently, and more predictably with the proper treatment or under optimal conditions. The idea has a certain appealing logic to it—the notion that "If you've done it once, you can do it again." Certainly the best treatment data suggest that this is true.

Patients who do not display these characteristics have a much bleaker prognosis that may become even more bleak as time post onset progresses. Those with the poorest prognoses are patients who are medically and neurologically stable at 1 month post onset, whose predicted overall percentile may be significantly above their present overall score, but who exhibit very little variation of item scores or modality scores.

The single best predictor of eventual recovery may be the patient's performance on a standardized language test at 1 month post onset. Yet there are other factors to consider, many of which are not as easily quantifiable. They include (1) inability to participate in treatment (e.g., inability to respond to any test items or test materials); (2) consistent inability to retain learned responses for 24 hours despite intensive drill and reinforcement; (3) plateaus maintained over periods of weeks with no gains or only minimal gains; and (4) agreement that the patient could get along as well or better outside of the hospital and continue to improve (Schuell et al., 1964). Schuell and associates presented a bleak picture of prognosis: "The only real objection is the amount of clinical time required to reach conclusions that are now predictable as soon as patients are neurologically stable" (p. 303). What they suggested is that a great deal about eventual recovery levels in aphasia is known from data obtained at 1 month post onset. What is yet to be discovered is how significant, in terms of functional recovery, that unexplained variance is, and how that potential can best be enhanced—in a sense, making clinicians poorer prognosticators.

In the author's clinic, a number of variables analyzed collectively have been found to foreshadow eventual recovery. These are discussed in the next section, where those factors that suggest poor, fair, and good prognosis for recovery are grouped for each category.

## SUMMARY PROFILES

### Poor Prognosis for Recovery

#### Medical Data

Usually the cause is a large lesion of the left hemisphere, compromising both the frontal and temporal lobes, of thrombolic or embolic origin, and usually greater than 100 cm$^3$. A severe right hemiplegia usually accompanies this lesion, as well as a right homonymous hemianopsia.

#### Language Data

**Porch Index of Communicative Ability (PICA.)** Performance on the PICA will be well below the 25th percentile at 1 month post onset, and will probably be nearer the 10th. Overall variability may be misleadingly high, but most scores will be very low, nearer 100, and no one modality will be strikingly better than another. Imitation, copying, and matching will usually be somewhat better. When the magnitude of these differences is not great, more fine-grained analysis is appropriate. Variance may be revealed only within subtests. Performance on these subtests may be significantly better than other modalities, but the mean subtest scores will not reach 15.

A PICA score (Fig. 4–1) placed him at the 3rd percentile for aphasic adults. He was awake, alert, and responsive. Overall variability (131) and

**Porch Index of Communicative Ability**

SCORE SHEET

Name III-A-391 Onset 5-21-85 No. 1

Date 6-18-85 By MJC Time 10:51 to 11:38 Total Time

Test Conditions STANDARD

Patient Conditions GOOD

Glasses: N Hearing aid: N Dentures: N Hand Used: (L)

| ITEM | I | II | III | IV | V | VI | VII | VIII | IX | X | XI | XII | A | B | C | D | E | F |
|---|---|---|---|---|---|---|---|---|---|---|---|---|---|---|---|---|---|---|
| 1. Tb | 2 | 2 | 2 | 2 | 6 | 2 | 6 | 6 | 3 | 6 | 15 | 4 | 5 | 5 | 5 | 5 | 4 | 6 |
| 2. Cg | 2 | 2 | 2 | 2 | 6 | 2 | 6 | 7 | 3 | 7 | 15 | 3 | 5 | 5 | 5 | 5 | 6 | 4 |
| 3. Pn | 2 | 2 | 2 | 2 | 6 | 2 | 7 | 13 | 3 | 2 | 15 | 3 | 5 | 5 | 5 | 5 | 4 | 4 |
| 4. Kf | 2 | 2 | 2 | 2 | 6 | 2 | 6 | 6 | 3 | 6 | 14 | 3 | 5 | 5 | 5 | 5 | 4 | 4 |
| 5. Fk | 2 | 2 | 2 | 2 | 6 | 2 | 6 | 13 | 3 | 6 | 13 | 3 | 5 | 5 | 5 | 5 | 4 | 4 |
| 6. Qt | 2 | 2 | 2 | 2 | 6 | 2 | 6 | 6 | 3 | 6 | 15 | 3 | 5 | 5 | 5 | 5 | 4 | 4 |
| 7. Pl | 2 | 2 | 2 | 2 | 6 | 2 | 6 | 13 | 3 | 6 | 15 | 3 | 5 | 5 | 5 | 5 | 4 | 4 |
| 8. Mt | 2 | 2 | 2 | 2 | 6 | 2 | 6 | 6 | 3 | 6 | 13 | 3 | 5 | 5 | 5 | 5 | 4 | 4 |
| 9. Ky | 2 | 2 | 2 | 2 | 6 | 2 | 6 | 6 | 3 | 9 | 13 | 3 | 5 | 5 | 5 | 5 | 4 | 4 |
| 10. Cb | 2 | 2 | 2 | 2 | 6 | 2 | 6 | 13 | 3 | 6 | 15 | 3 | 5 | 5 | 5 | 5 | 4 | 4 |
| TIME | :56 | :00 | :03 | :07 | :10 | :14 | :16 | :17 | :18 | :22 | :24 | :26 | :29 | :31 | :33 | :35 | :37 | :39 |
| MINUTES | 5 | 4 | 3 | 4 | 3 | 4 | 1 | 1 | 1 | 4 | 2 | 3 | 2 | 2 | 2 | 2 | 2 | 2 |
| MODALITY | VRB | PTM | PTM | VRB | RDG | AUD | RDG | VIS | VRB | AUD | VIS | VRB | WRI | WRI | WRI | WRI | CPY | CPY |
| MEAN SCORE | 2.0 | 2.0 | 2.0 | 2.0 | 6.0 | 2.0 | 6.1 | 8.9 | 3.0 | 6.0 | 14.4 | 3.1 | 5.0 | 5.0 | 5.0 | 5.0 | 4.2 | 4.2 |
| %ILE | 0/1 | 0/1 | 0/1 | 0/1 | 15 | 0/1 | 11 | 3 | 2/5 | 3 | 11 | 4 | 20 | 16 | 16 | 15 | 7 | 2 |
| VARIAB. | 1 | 1 | 1 | 1 | 1 | 1 | 9 | 41 | 1 | 30 | 6 | 9 | 1 | 1 | 1 | 1 | 18 | 18 |

| MPO | OVERALL | WRITING | COPYING | READING | PANTOMIME | VERBAL | AUDITORY | VISUAL |
|---|---|---|---|---|---|---|---|---|
| 1 | 4.77 | 5.00 | 4.20 | 6.05 | 2.00 | 2.53 | 4.00 | 11.65 |
| %ile | 3 | 20 | 3 | 12 | 1 | 1 | 1 | 4 |
| Variab. | 131 | 0 | 36 | 9 | 0 | 9 | 30 | 47 |
| Mean Var. | 7.3 | 0 | 18.00 | 4.50 | 0 | 2.30 | 15.00 | 23.5 |

| | Gestural | Verbal | Graphic | 9 HI | 9 LO | HOAP | Correction | Target |
|---|---|---|---|---|---|---|---|---|
| Score | 5.92 | 2.53 | 4.73 | 6.82 | 2.72 | 5.92 | | |
| %ile | 2 | 1 | 3 | 4 | 1 | 9th | | 9th %ile |

CONSULTING PSYCHOLOGISTS PRESS
577 College Avenue Palo Alto, California

**Figure 4–1.** PICA score sheet for a patient with poor potential for recovery.

mean variability suggest an extremely poor prognosis and, in fact, his projected performance at 6 months post onset is at the 9th percentile.

Most alarming was his 3rd percentile rank for matching pictures to objects, objects to objects, and copying. The ability to copy a few words or a few letters, or the ability to match a few objects, does not suggest that functional language competence will return, but accurate performance on a few of these tasks is usually a prelude to some recovery. On all verbal tests, even those requiring "yes" and "no," the patient's responses were unintelligible, undifferentiated monosyllables that were occasionally strung together for several repetitions.

**Other Tests.** Performance on the BDAE will yield no distinctive pattern of preserved components. Mean auditory comprehension will be well below the 25th percentile, and aphasia severity rating will be 1. The WAB will yield an AQ of 0 to 37.6, again with no discernible pattern of preserved components.

Performance on the *Token Test* will be below 15 of 61 correct. Performance on the *Reading Comprehension Battery for Aphasia* will be between 5 and 10 correct (of 30 possible) on the first three subtests, a distinct decline in performance after that, and overall performance below 30 correct. On Raven's *Coloured Progressive Matrices* (RCPM), performance will rarely exceed 15 of 36 correct, and more often 5 to 10 correct is achieved.

Nonstandard assessment (e.g., on the Mayo Clinic *Procedures for Language Evaluation* [MAYO]) will reflect preserved abilities far more sensitively. Even patients with a poor prognosis will follow one or two personal commands; produce several numbers in sequence to imitation; complete an occasional, high probability sentence (e.g., "The flag is red, white, and *blue*"); or even approximate copies of single letters and words. This test will reveal few abilities beyond these.

Performance on the oral, nonverbal, and limb apraxia batteries will probably yield no correct responses on request, perhaps one or two to repetition, and as many as several correct responses to imitation.

Appropriate responses to the series of yes-no questions presented in Chapter 3 will occasionally be given. Patients who give equivocal responses and recurring utterances and who are unable to indicate a clear "yes" or "no" have a poorer prognosis.

A series of environmental questions (e.g., "Do you have the time?", "Did you bring your glasses with you?", or "Where's your wedding ring?") and contrived artifices (e.g., presenting the patient with a book turned upside down, or with an empty cup) will often brighten the eyes and responses of most globally aphasic patients. Their failure to respond to more than one or two of these will dim the bright eyes of even the most enthusiastic clinician. For patients with the poorest prognoses, testing even at this level will yield few appropriate responses.

The most eloquent evidence of what will become a chronic, global aphasia is a flat performance profile with little variation over several days or sessions and a demonstrated inability to learn even the simplest tasks, despite numerous demonstrations and repetitions. The time required for complete diagnostic testing will be considerable. A simple, relatively inexpensive measure that can be administered over several days or sessions might consist of a 10 item copying task, an imitation task, or a series of biographical questions requiring "yes" and "no" responses.

At 6 months post onset, this patient had reached his predicted recovery level. There were no bright spots in his performance. Although he appeared to recognize familiar places and faces, laughed appropriately, and was responsive and attentive, his communicative abilities improved little.

## Fair Prognosis for Recovery

### Medical Data

Usually results from a large lesion of the left hemisphere, but lesion size is not much greater than 100 cm$^3$.

### Language Testing

Patients with a fair prognosis for recovery will display some promise on comprehensive tests of communicative ability. Performance on the PICA will be below the 25th percentile, but there will be more disparity among modality scores and more variability among and within subtests. Total variability will be well above 100. The ability to copy accurately if not well, to match most objects correctly, to name or approximate the name of one or two objects, and to produce differentiated but unintelligible responses on the verbal subtests foreshadows a fair prognosis. A PICA score sheet for a patient with a fair prognosis is shown in Figure 4-2. Although overall performance is very low, six of ten items on the auditory subtests are correct, although the patient required a cue for the correct response on one. On another item the patient self-corrected, suggesting good capacity for monitoring his responses. The ability to self-correct in severely aphasic patients, particularly in the early stages of recovery, fosters optimism in even the most pessimistic clinician. This patient also had five correct responses on the reading subtests and made three related errors, all of which suggest potential for recovery.

BDAE severity score may be 1 but is more likely to be 2. Performance on auditory comprehension subtests will be above the 15th percentile and nearer the 25th. WAB aphasia quotients will hover near 25, and a profile of deficits will reveal the beginnings of a pattern of preserved components.

Performance on the *Token Test* will be nearer 15; on the RCPM performance will probably not be significantly better than 15, but it may be near 20.

Nonstandard assessments including the MAYO will reveal some preserved components, including the ability both to produce several serials of each type and to follow a few commands.

Early impressions of this patient's potential for recovery were realized. His recovery level at 6 months post onset, based on HOAP scores, was projected to the 15th percentile. That dire prognosis was tempered, however, because of the potential he showed on more difficult subtests of the PICA; his relatively high variability; his responsiveness in conversational, spontaneous situations; and his occasional ability to self-correct. Because these factors could not be weighted, the prognosis was not entirely objective. Fortunately, patients know little about objective test results, and this patient cared less. His performance eventually reached the 47th percentile.

## Good Prognosis for Recovery

### Medical Data

Usually a much smaller lesion of the left hemisphere. As a general rule, the smaller and more circumscribed the lesion, the better the prognosis is for recovery.

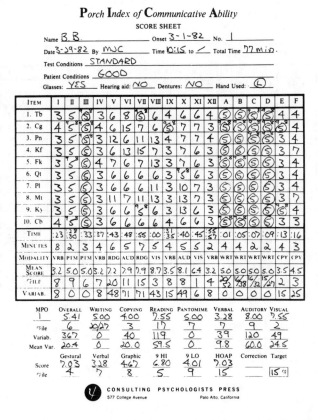

**Figure 4–2.** PICA score sheet for a patient with fair potential for recovery.

### Language Testing

Performance on the PICA will be nearer an overall score of 8 but still well below the 25th percentile, with significant peaks of performance, and several scores of "7" and higher on auditory comprehension, reading, and naming subtests. Variability will be much greater than in the two previous examples. In Figure 4–3, variability is shown above 400, even though overall performance is at the 9th percentile. Overall variability is not as potent a prediction variable in this example as it is an examination of patterns of variability. On the auditory, verbal, and pantomime modalities, variability is very high (95, 71, and 89, respectively);

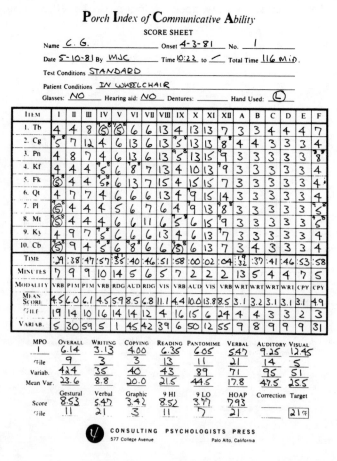

**Figure 4–3.** PICA score sheet for a patient with good potential for recovery.

it is much lower in other areas. Because these subtests are generally more difficult for aphasic patients, the patient's frequent ability to perform them correctly (15 of 20 correct on the auditory subtests, for example) is striking, and suggests excellent potential.

The patient's performance on other language tests will be correspondingly higher. Limb and oral, nonverbal apraxia may not be a potent predictor, and visual, nonverbal problem-solving ability is likely to be variable.

This particular patient recovered to the 76th percentile 1 year after his stroke. If predictions based on comparisons to a large sample of aphasic individuals had been used, such recovery would have seemed impossible. The examination of other objective variables, however, suggested his potential. This example does succumb to subjectivity but the subjective impressions are based on objective data.

## SUMMARY

This chapter has presented summaries of a number of measures for the formal and informal assessment of aphasia. The battery is admittedly a biased one and a reflection of the author's experience and training. Readers may wish to administer a different combination of tests or different tests entirely. The tests, however, should compromise between brevity and exhaustiveness and should allow both the selection of the most appropriate treatment goals and techniques and a reasonably accurate prediction of the patient's response to treatment and physiological recovery.

The author admits that these tests fall far short of total objectivity. That they come close at all is a tribute to current knowledge about the aphasic patient. The tests' occasionally inaccurate estimates of eventual recovery and response to treatment should prompt clinicians not to abandon them but to improve them.

Of course performance of the measures discussed here will be variable, both within and among patients. This variability will depend on a host of factors, including the severity of the aphasia, the time of day, presence of depression, recency of onset, medications, medical conditions, and the patient's enthusiasm. The summary of scores shown in Table 4–1, however, reflects the general range of performance of globally aphasic patients on selected speech and language tasks.

**Table 4–1.  Summary of Diagnostic Performance Variables in Global Aphasia**

| Assessment | Severity |
| --- | --- |
| *General Communicative Ability* | |
| PICA | |
| Overall Score | 3.15–8.38 |
| Overall Percentile | 1st–25th |
| Total Variability | 0–300 |
| BDAE | |
| Aphasia Severity | 1 |
| Auditory Comprehension | 1st–25th |
| WAB | |
| Aphasia Quotient | 0–37.6 |
| Fluency | 0–4 |
| Comprehension | 0–3.9 |
| Repetition | 0–4.9 |
| Naming | 0–6 |
| *Reading* | |
| Reading Comprehension Battery for Aphasia | |
| Total Score | 0–30 |
| Word Recognition with One Foil | |
| Personally Salient Stimuli | 0–50% |
| *Auditory Comprehension* | |
| Token Test Total Score | 0–13 |
| Yes-No Questions | |
| Personal | 0–40% |
| Environmental | 0–30% |
| Informational | 0–30% |
| Following Directions | |
| Body | 0–50% |
| Nonbody | 0–30% |
| *Speaking* | |
| Boston Naming Test | 0–6 |
| Serial Speech | None to variable for counting 1–10, several days of the week, a few letters |
| Repetition | Some single words, rarely sentences. |
| Sentence Completion | None to several (high probability) |
| *Writing* | |
| Copying | None to a few single letters and words, name |
| Spontaneous | Generally no intelligible writing |

*Apraxia Battery*
  Request                                                 0–4
  Repetition                                     0–6
  Imitation                                      0–8

*Cognitive Abilities*
  Coloured Progressive Matrices Total Score          0–20, generally 15 or below

# Chapter 5

# General Considerations and Techniques in the Management of the Globally Aphasic Patient

## HISTORICAL PERSPECTIVES

Darley (1979) has done much to make aphasiologists feel good about what they do: "We do not depend upon sentiment or intuition in declaring that therapy works. It works so well that every neurologist, physiatrist, and speech-language pathologist responsible for patient management should refuse to accede to a plan that abandons the patient to neglect" (p. 629). Darley's extraordinarily optimistic statement sustains us, but despite his assurances, many clinicians are timid about their ability to help, and global aphasia provides a substantial challenge. Schuell and associates (1964) as well as others added their support with data and their convictions.

Schuell and colleagues in particular have provided a bleak picture of the globally aphasic patient's future: "The characteristic of Group Five patients is not that they make no gains but that gains do not become functional" (p. 305). That, it seems, is the heart of the issue. All treatment, at some level, is effective. Clinicians may be sanguine, for example, about the ability of imitation tasks to elicit imitation, the effects of copying to elicit copying, and the effects of matching to elicit matching. They can even feel secure in the knowledge that patients can imitate, copy, and match more difficult stimuli in some sort of hierarchical fashion as treatment progresses. These skills, however, do not necessarily precede functional communication skills.

Communication is the ability to convey thoughts, desires, attitudes, and needs. Imitation, matching, and copying do not permit communication in these terms, yet they do have value. They set the stage for further treatment by introducing structured treatment tasks, they may become the foundation of functional communication, and they allow the clinician to gain insight into skills and deficits that cannot be obtained in any other way. Clinicians believe in this rationale because they have observed its effects. But because they have no empirical evidence to support their conclusions, the value of treatment at this level is viewed with some skepticism by other professionals. Perhaps this is fair. It may also be, however, that a more rigorous examination of these procedures will demonstrate their worth.

This section on treatment will reflect the premise that globally aphasic patients can learn a number of skills, including matching, copying, and imitation, but the primary justification for training patients in these skills is to pursue a course leading to more functional skills. The skills should function as diagnostic tools in an expanded diagnostic repertoire, as warm-up tasks, and as necessary precursors to the more demanding treatment tasks required for functional communication. There are other tasks that seem to serve the same function.

Visual action therapy (Helm and Benson, 1978) is often extolled as a precursor to other treatment tasks, and it may accomplish some of these goals better than copying, matching, and imitating. There is no evidence that visual action therapy is more effective than other tasks, however. The treatments described in this chapter include a number of tasks that do not necessarily lead to functional communication. They are included not because they allow the clinician to fill up the clinical hour with rewarding activities but because they are preliminaries to functional communication training. In general, the clinical philosophy is "If it isn't broke, don't fix it." The following discussion centers on using residual language and alternative (often innovative) strategies, building on these abilities to improve communication but not necessarily to improve language.

## ENVIRONMENTAL TREATMENT

Lubinski (1981) states that one of the responsibilities of clinicians is to help establish a positive communicative environment. Her strategies for doing that, which are particularly appropriate for the globally aphasic patient, include facing the patient; alerting the patient that communication is about to occur; speaking slowly and clearly in "adult talk"; talking about concrete topics; keeping related topics together; using short, syntactically complete utterances; pausing between utterances;

and using nonverbal cues to augment communication. These general considerations provide a positive therapeutic milieu for the procedures that will follow.

## Controlling the Environment

Other factors that may have a negative influence on the communicative environment include the following:

1. *Posture.* Hemiplegic patients, especially those confined to a wheelchair, frequently are uncomfortable. Because their involved side does not provide adequate support, they lean to that side. Leaning increases the pressure on extremities on the involved side, and an uncomfortable patient will not be as responsive. Positioning—and often repositioning—to improve a patient's posture will help ensure that a patient's attention is on the treatment and not on his discomfort.

2. *Positioning.* The patient should be positioned so that his or her view of the therapy materials or of the therapist is unobstructed; avoid placing an additional burden on the patient by making it necessary for him or her to assume an awkward posture to see or reach the treatment materials. Face-to-face is generally the most effective position, but some clinicians prefer to sit on the patient's nonhemiplegic side.

Homonymous hemianopsia is common in global aphasia, and controlling for its effects is relatively simple. Materials should be placed to the left of midline and, depending on whether the hemianopsia includes the upper or lower quadrant, slightly above or below the usual line of vision. To ensure that patients can see all materials, ask him or her to look at all the materials on the perimeter. If a patient consistently attends only to the involved (usually the left) side, it may be through neglect, but it is more likely because of the hemianopsia.

## Emotion, Anger, and Grieving

Globally aphasic patients—like all other people—have a right to emotional release. Grieving and depression are natural responses to devastating illness, and global aphasia does not make an individual immune to despair. Patients react bitterly to the blow caused by their illness, and they may respond angrily to the condition they are so powerless to change. As will be seen in a later section, there are times when fragile psyches require that treatment be forestalled. Patients may need time to adjust, but they usually get on with the task and with life.

The clinician must recognize that grieving is part of healing, and although it may interfere with treatment, it should not prevent treatment. The clinician should be empathic and respond with appropriate gestures, an occasional pat, an appropriately soothing verbal response, and an attitude of clear acceptance and understanding. The chronically emotionally labile patient is the exception rather than the rule. Control of emotional responses, and the ability to inhibit these responses, is probably a combination of physiological recovery and acceptance of the individual's deficits. An atmosphere of acceptance, but with continued focus on the task at hand, will eventually establish the conditions for effective treatment.

Depression is a natural consequence of stroke, and few clinicians blame aphasic patients for experiencing depression. The difficulty of studying depression in aphasia, however, has generally prevented adequate assessment. Fromm, Holland, and Swindell (1984) documented the nature and course of early depression in 59 left hemisphere damaged stroke patients and examined the relationship between depression and other variables, including speech and language.

Fromm and colleagues (1984) found that 31 percent of the entire left hemisphere stroke group was mildly to moderately depressed. Of the aphasic group, 48 percent were mildly to moderately depressed. These authors also found a significant relationship between final Aphasia Quotient (AQ) and depression score. Although type of aphasia had no significant effect, living situation (nursing home) and recovery (not recovered by 2 months post onset) were significant variables that yielded higher proportions of depressed patients.

Several important implications arise from this study. First, depression is apparently a frequent (and appropriate) response to stroke, and may play a significant role in recovery. Second, living situation appears to have a significant influence on depression. Generally, the more independent the patient the more likely he or she is to return to the same premorbid living situation. Independence in communication is a significant factor in determining eventual placement. Ensuring some communicative independence is incumbent on the speech-language pathologist. Third, globally aphasic patients are more likely to be depressed, and their depression is likely to be more severe. Overcoming, or at least recognizing, that depression will play an important part in treating that patient's speech and language deficits.

Finally, it should be remembered that depression is treatable. Language deficits generally preclude traditional psychotherapy, but excellent relief from the symptoms of depression have been obtained using short-term antidepressants (Ross and Rush, 1981). Failure to thrive in treatment may be related to depression and is at least a hypothesis worth testing.

## GROUP TREATMENT

Group treatment for aphasia has been both condemned (Schuell et al., 1964) and extolled (Wertz et al., 1981). With the exception of Wertz and colleagues and Aten, Caligiuri, and Holland (1980), evidence for efficacy of group treatment is mostly anecdotal. The two studies cited, however, found significant effects from group treatment. Wertz and associates found that group treatment and individual treatment were about equally efficacious. Aten and colleagues found that chronically aphasic patients, who were no longer making measurable gains from individual treatment, made significant gains after 3 months of group treatment. The objective evidence, then, is in favor of group treatment, and it is surprising that more clinicians do not practice it, or that more patients are not given the opportunity to benefit from it.

Group treatment might be particularly appropriate for globally aphasic patients because they possess adequate social skills. West, in Aten et al. (1981), found that severely aphasic patients, although they have a more difficult time within a group structure, can do quite well in the group setting. She emphasizes visual aids, finds that the group is maximally supportive, and with these visual aids finds that the severely aphasic patient can usually be integrated into the group structure.

Marquardt, Tonkovich, and DeVault (1976) state that group therapy should be structured to meet a triad of goals—speech, sociotherapeutic, and psychotherapeutic. To meet these general goals, the focus of group therapy may be direct, in (1) providing a continuation or extension of speech and language training similar in content to that done in individual sessions or (2) providing a transfer medium for speech and language usage with more than just the individual treatment therapist. The focus may be indirect, with the more general goals of experiencing speaking and listening with other patients who have similar problems, under which circumstances the demands for exact communication supposedly are reduced. Groups may also have alternative objectives—for example, identifying inappropriate social greeting responses and modifying these in the actual social setting of a group, or perhaps helping patients begin a communicative utterance with the appropriate pronoun.

Socialization may be the most traditional and common objective of groups. Socialization is more fun than traditional, direct activities and it provides contact and interactions for patients which they might not otherwise have. Examples of group socialization activities might include lectures, group outings to sporting events, games of chance based on films of horse races, and field trips.

Haire (in Aten et al., 1981) described an intensive group treatment program at Memphis State University. The overall objective of this program (which included one half hour of small group therapy, one half hour of social activities, and one hour of large group activities) is to help the patient to maximize his or her communicative strengths to improve interpersonal interactions, either as part of the carry-over process from individual treatment or as an extension of the speech and language training done in individual treatment.

The groups are task oriented. That is, the interactions center on a task or a game that is preplanned by the clinician. These tasks are based on five basic principles:

1. The task should be conducive to using communicative patterns that will encourage group interactions. This principle is facilitated by encouraging the patient to interact by assisting, supporting, giving feedback, questioning, and arguing.
2. The task should provide the patient with an opportunity to communicate with success, and the patient should have the freedom to communicate through any modality he or she chooses.
3. The task should be structured so that there is decreasing dependence on the clinician. If possible, communication should be spontaneous rather than clinician-directed.
4. A motivator should be incorporated into the group—for example, one chosen from the patient's history or current interests.
5. The task should be kept simple.

The difficulty of measuring progress in group treatment has been addressed but not resolved. Because the focus is on communication and socialization, not on the improvement of language, improvement in the former areas is not likely to be revealed by traditional tests. Davis and Wilcox (1981) have proposed a speech act analysis of aphasic communication in group settings that seems promising. Wertz and colleagues (1981) used a weekly checklist for their patients in group treatment. Ten behaviors (five activity-related and five language-related) were rated. The five activity-related behaviors were the following:

1. Did the patient attend to the activity?
2. Was the patient's behavior appropriate to the task?
3. Did the patient participate in the activity without clinician assistance?
4. Did the patient follow through on suggestions given?
5. Did the patient generate ideas for future activities?

The five language-related behaviors were the following:

1. Did the patient attend to what others said?
2. Did the patient follow the main ideas expressed by others?
3. Did the patient initiate communication without clinician direction?
4. Were the patient's responses appropriate to the topic?
5. Did the patient communicate ideas in a clear manner?

All behaviors were rated on a scale of 1 to 5 (1 indicating "never," 5 indicating "normal").

The general treatment principles for group treatment used in this study were far-ranging. They were designed to enhance the patient's communicative abilities without direct manipulation of speech and language, with emphasis on stimulating communicative skills through group socialization, peer interaction and support, participation of members in activities relative to their interests and needs, and nondirective stimulation from the clinician. Emphasis was placed on communication of ideas and problem-solving tasks, and the sessions included exploration of personal and family adjustment problems, general intellectual stimulation (for example, discussion of current events), and activities of specific interest to members of the group or the group as a whole. Specific methodology included the following:

1. Treatment activities were selected to tax, but not to exceed, the communicative abilities of the patients in the group.
2. Treatment included content-centered discussions, which the therapist conducted, and topics were selected by group members or the therapist.
3. Treatment included problem-solving through role-playing.
4. Treatment was supplemented, complemented, or extended by activities not requiring the presence of the clinician (for example, films, educational lectures, community projects).
5. In general, the clinician was encouraged to suggest activities appropriate for the group, encourage participation of each group member at appropriate levels of response complexity, summarize group discussions, provide reinforcement for participation in group activities, encourage expression of attitudes and feelings, and encourage communication among group members.

Treatment activities for these groups, which ranged in size from three to seven persons, included combinations of the following:

1. Group discussions of topics of current interest.
2. Creative activities, such as painting, model building, and so forth.

3.  Recreational activities, such as cards and other games, contests, and so forth.
4.  Role-playing of problem situations.
5.  Individual reports or talks by group members dealing with current events, experiences, problems, and similar topics.
6.  Invited talks or presentations by outside persons on subjects of interest to the group; community resources, services, or facilities; and rehabilitation information.

Supplementary activities consisted of the following:

1.  Attendance at films, plays, concerts, lectures, and similar events.
2.  Participation in athletic activities, such as bowling and swimming.
3.  Participation in community activities or projects.
4.  Hobby activities, such as painting, stamp collecting, and weaving.
5.  Participation in group excursions and tours.
6.  Problem-solving puzzles and games.

For more specific group activities, the reader is directed to the works by Aten and colleagues (1981), Bloom (1962), Wilcox and Davis (1977), and Marquardt and associates (1976).


## COUNSELING THE FAMILY

Counseling the family of a patient with aphasia takes many forms; its content will depend on the family, their needs, their knowledge of the disorder, and their willingness to accept that counseling. The family's response to this devastating illness are rarely predictable, at least to clinicians unfamiliar with them, and counseling should begin gently and tentatively.

The family's first questions are usually about the stroke itself: what happened, why did it happen, will it happen again, when will the patient get better? The best medical personnel make themselves available to answer these questions, and they are the best ones to answer those questions. Frequently, however, the burden falls to speech-language clinicians. Aphasiologists are not a bad choice for the role of answering questions; they know a great deal about the causes, the disease process, and the aftermath of stroke. Several precautions are appropriate for clinicians in the situation.

First, they are not medical people and should not assume responsibilities for talking about medications, medical treatment, or recovery from hemiplegia. Specific questions about stroke and its physical aftermath should be answered by trained medical personnel and augmented by available literature. The primary role of aphasiologists here is to serve as the primary source of information about the disruption of speech and language in aphasia. It is prudent, however, to first review the patient's medical chart carefully to avoid misinterpreting and misinforming the family about the patient.

Counseling should not be limited to a single encounter but should unfold as the family's understanding of the patient's deficits evolves. Families are not usually ready for the hard questions initially, and neither are clinicians. It is good to try to meet with the family at least several times: at the beginning of treatment, sometime after they have had a chance to absorb the information given to them, during treatment, and again before the patient is discharged from the hospital, or before treatment is terminated. The families of some patients seem to require daily contact with the people providing care. In many cases clinicians become their communicative lifeline to the patient. This support is reciprocated, because families are the best source for learning about the effects of treatment and for deciding on treatment goals.

Aphasiologists in general are not trained to deal with family dynamics, particularly potentially explosive ones. If the situation warrants it, professional counseling, perhaps with the clinician serving as interpreter or resource, is often useful, and counseling is available in many hospitals and clinics.

As the aphasia evolves, and as the spouse's knowledge of the disorder and the patient's deficits grows, questions frequently become more specific. Because the trauma has lessened, clinicians usually feel freer to talk more specifically about deficits or about the very real possibility that there will be no return to work or an unfettered retirement, as had long been planned. The rehabilitation team becomes, or should become, a unified group at this point, and counseling may be more effective when it takes the form of panel discussions with the patient or family, or both, as participants.

In summary, counseling for the family may be nearly as important as treatment (or may not be separated from treatment) for the globally aphasic patient. It helps reduce the impact of aphasia and to uncover some of its mysteries, and, by doing so, makes the topic more approachable. In the best of situations, it prepares the family to provide a positive, supportive communicative environment to allow the best expression of the patient's communicative skills. It should continue, formally or informally, as long as the therapeutic relationship exists.

## Bibliotherapy

Bibliotherapy is not an appropriate counseling technique for every family, but the best of the written materials provide reassurance and instruction that often cannot be obtained in a personal encounter. Families can take these resources with them, unlike much of the information clinicians can provide, which although abundant makes only a fleeting impression in the clinic. Sarno's *Stroke* (1963) is an excellent example, and Boone (1965) presents the complex topic of aphasia in a forthright and understandable manner. A list of these sources and others appears at the end of this chapter.

## Stroke Clubs

Stroke clubs seem to fill a need for many stroke patients and their families and caregivers. The number of members in the United States is unknown, but according to Sanders, Hamby, and Nelson (1984) there are at least 302 clubs or sponsors in the United States alone. The structure, focus, and membership profiles of the clubs vary, but they provide support that would otherwise be unavailable to many stroke patients and their families.

The American Heart Association will provide information concerning stroke clubs according to geographical location in addition to information on forming new clubs. The address of this organization is given in Appendix 6-1.

## EDUCATING STAFF MEMBERS

Global aphasia is not new to most hospital rehabilitation staff members but, like most people, they need occasional reminders to remember what they do know. For example, the staff members may need to be reminded that globally aphasic patients do not understand everything they hear, despite their knowing nods and their growing recognition and learning of daily hospital routine. Infrequently they may need to be reminded that the globally aphasic patient does not need to be treated like a child, that a severe hearing loss is not usually part of the problem, and that alphabet boards are likely to be as effective a device for communicating with globally aphasic patients as Hindi is for a midwesterner. Such attitudes are as dangerous to a patient as the assumption that he or she knows when to take medication or knows how to get from the speech department to the physical therapy department because the ward secretary gave him or her directions.

The staff members should be as fully informed about the patient's condition as aphasiologists can make them. Inform them through reports of evaluation, through weekly or more frequent staff meetings, through in-service meetings on aphasia and related disorders, and through reminders about how best to communicate with the globally aphasic patient. These suggestions are as valuable to the staff members as they are to the patient and family because they help extend the positive communicative environment clinicians provide in 1 or 2 hours of daily treatment. Clinicians know that time is not enough. Realizing that, and capitalizing on the very sincere desire of the staff members to help and to rehabilitate, will do as much for treatment effects and generalization as the most potent treatment stimuli.

## Guidelines for Communicating with the Severely or Globally Aphasic Patient

The following guidelines for communicating with a severely aphasic patient are grounded in common sense, at least to clinicians. The guidelines do not require a deep understanding of the nature of the deficit in global aphasia or special expertise in communication. They are as useful to the clinician to remember and use as they are for the staff members and the patient's family.

To begin with, it is best to operate at the least complex level and to keep your speech very simple while providing the maximum of clues. Patients should respond with "yes" or "no" answers. More specific guidelines include the following:

1. *Simplify.* Handle only one idea at a time; use short sentences with simple, common words; speak more slowly, but naturally; and do not speak to the patient as if he or she were a child.

2. *Clue the patient in.* Be sure you have the patient's attention; use gestures and pointing when possible; facial cues may also help the patient. Use redundant wording; for example, "Are you hungry enough to eat dinner?" Repeat and reword the idea until the patient understands.

3. *Allow time.* Allow the patient additional time to understand and to respond, and be patient, unhurried, and accepting of his or her speech attempts.

4. *Guess.* Determine the subject by asking increasingly specific questions. Make statements about what you think the patient means to make sure you understand.

5. *Confirm.* When the patient responds to a question, ask the opposite also. If the response does not change, you and the patient are not communicating.

6. *Be clear.* Say "I'm sorry, I don't understand you" when necessary. Do not leave abruptly when attempts fail.

7. *Reduce extraneous variables.* Such variables include a noisy environment, additional activities such as television or radio, and talking with more than one person at a time.

8. *Respect.* The patient is usually an intelligent adult who is quite aware of his or her surroundings even though language function is impaired. Include the patient in the conversation; do not treat him or her as if he or she were not there or were deaf or mentally retarded.

These suggestions are critically important because they help ensure that a patient's dignity is preserved and that communicative interactions are as natural as the patient's deficits and a sensitive listener will permit.

Because not every patient has the same set of symptoms or responds identically to environmental cues or facilitative strategies, and because clinicians cannot supervise every communicative interaction, they should not limit their influence to the patient's family, room, or hospital ward. It is effective to attach an abbreviated list of individualized suggestions for each patient to his or her wheelchair or the cover of the hospital chart. Much as an accompanying letter explaining a patient's condition might prevent the indignity of arrest following a traffic accident, these suggestions may help circumvent personal efforts and misunderstandings.

## Communication Competence Training for Patients and Staff Members

Towey and Pettit (1980) have formalized a program to enhance communicative interactions for severely and globally aphasic patients. This program preceded their work on the CCEI with a report of a treatment program implemented in a rural rehabilitation hospital. In this program, the goals and responsibilities for rehabilitation are shared by the entire staff.

Towey and Pettit's treatment program (1980) for global aphasia emphasizes communicative competence in nonlinguistic areas, including eye contact, head nods, facial expressions, reciprocity of affect, physical proximity, and posture. Important verbal behaviors included in this program include the use of names and appropriate titles and emphatic verbal responses by the patient's auditor.

Towey and Pettit (1980) suggested that the speech pathologist train all staff members to identify a number of nonlinguistic responses that occur in communicative interactions. This is done through lectures, discussions, and observations of the patient's treatment program. Staff members are encouraged to identify, use, and facilitate each area of communicative competence. In one aspect of the program, staff members are videotaped in communicative interaction with the patient, and the tapes are then reviewed with the staff person to identify thoughts and feelings experienced during the interactions.

Towey and Pettit (1980) believe that the key to improving the quality of life and ability to interact and function on a daily basis for globally aphasic patients rests in nonlinguistic treatment areas rather than intensive treatment that focuses on linguistic parameters. Accordingly, the central feature of this program involves training the staff members to identify these linguistic and nonlinguistic responses in communication interactions and to refine and facilitate the use of these responses in realistic communication situations. Each nursing staff member participates in a lecture discussion and observation program under the supervision of the speech-language pathologist to enhance his or her ability to identify, use, and facilitate each of the nine areas of communication competence. Part of this training is done through the use of videotaped recordings of a staff member interacting with a globally aphasic patient. The tapes are then reviewed by the staff person and a speech pathologist to identify thoughts and feelings experienced during the interactions, to increase empathic communication skills.

Rather than concentrate on direct approaches to improve traditional communication modalities, this program focuses on communication only peripherally at first. It capitalizes on the nonverbal skills that are intact, reinforcing and refining those skills through empathic modeling, and establishing a positive communicative environment. Many of these features are overlooked in other treatment programs and are worth recounting here.

**Names.** Through an interview with family and friends, the speech pathologist should determine the name or title the patient prefers (for example, Doctor, Professor, or Mrs.).

**Verbal Responses.** Verbal responses (for example, "I know that makes you angry") are used to indicate empathy. Listeners are also urged to avoid interrupting the speaker by attending to all aspects of the communication, by maintaining eye contact, and by avoiding distractions.

**Presence or Absence and Rate of Head Nods.** Listeners should indicate participation, understanding, and desire to respond with appropriate head nods. Slow head nodding, they say, may indicate a relaxed and attentive listener, but increased speed of nods may indicate that the listener wants to speak or is becoming anxious or impatient.

**Facial Expression.** Facial expression may be used to convey feelings of concern or fear, support or empathy, for the speaker. They may also be used to assist in understanding the patient's intent.

**Physical Proximity.** Close physical proximity may be used to indicate support, comfort, and contact with the patient. Too little distance may be unsettling to the patient, but too much distance (greater than 5½ feet) may also create discomfort. Some feeling of physical "closeness" should be preserved without violating the patient's space.

**General Postural Cues.** Certain leg and foot movements during conversation may indicate anxiety or tranquility, participation or inattention.

Through a program that emphasized the positive aspects of each of these linguistic and nonverbal features, Towey and Pettit (1980) found that several globally aphasic patients made significant gains in communication skills, but not in linguistic skills.

## ESTABLISHING REALISTIC GOALS

Goals need not always be increment markers on a continuum, unless that continuum is viewed in a more philosophical, spiritual sense. As often as possible, however, the goals should be realistic and carefully planned, but with a willingness to be opportunistic and accepting when another avenue is revealed. Goals should not be predicated on the notion that the achievement of one goal necessarily means that a newer, more difficult goal is attainable.

The attainment of some goals should probably suggest a switch to another modality or working on maintaining that behavior, or alert the clinician to begin the process that leads to the termination of treatment. Deciding what the goals should be, and recognizing when these goals will yield to another level, or when they are unattainable, is a clinical art, as much intuition and insight as science.

Realistic goals should begin with a needs assessment. All patients need to communicate, but some patients feel the need more than others, and some patients are less dependent on speech. Part of our understanding of what the patient's needs are will come from data gathered in the clinical sessions, but we need also rely on the family interview and covert assessments of the patient.

Realistic goals for globally aphasic patients should proceed from the assumption that they possess fundamentally sound recognition skills that permit an awareness of, but limited interaction with, their environment. These skills do not require training. Although it may be a realistic and attainable goal, training the patient in these skills may have more value if tasks to enhance attention, resource allocation, and warm-up are emphasized rather than communication goals.

Realistic goals should begin with the basic communicative needs of the patient and coincide with those of the clinician and family. These goals should have a reasonable certainty of success. Examples of realistic goals include the following:

1.  Improving auditory comprehension, supplemented with contextual cues, to permit consistent comprehension of one-step commands in well-controlled situations.

2. Improving production to make "yes" and "no" consistent, unequivocal responses in controlled situations.
3. Improving ability to spontaneously produce several written responses, or approximations, of functional or salient words of daily living.
4. Improving production of several simple, unequivocal gestures.
5. Improving drawing so that several simple, unequivocal messages can be conveyed in this modality.
6. Ensuring that a small, basic core of communicative intentions can be conveyed in one or a combination of modalities.

It is realistic to expect that these goals can be attained. They should be minimal goals for all globally aphasic patients. Expanding this repertoire will depend on a number of factors, including the patient's availability for treatment, cooperation and motivation, and general health. Enhancing and improving on these goals may not always be possible. If new goals beckon, because a patient has demonstrated a capacity to reach them, they should be welcomed.

The preceding section included suggestions for establishing the conditions for creating a positive communicative environment. They deserve equal consideration and rank with the more specific techniques that are described in later chapters. They are appropriate not just for the globally aphasic patient but also for patients with less severe deficits. The most effective treatment goes beyond drill and detail, and assumes a responsibility for preserving that positive therapeutic environment outside the clinic walls.

*Chapter* **6**

# Treatment Considerations for the Globally Aphasic Patient

## ASSESSING TREATMENT FOR THE GLOBALLY APHASIC PATIENT

The treatment of globally aphasic patients should be scientifically rigorous, but the science should not overwhelm the treatment. That is, clinicians should not lose sight of the need to treat the patient, but they should be able to *demonstrate* both the need for treatment and the patient's response to treatment. Clinicians are frequently reminded of the need for adequate data to back up their treatment choices as a justification of their worth to other professionals and those who provide support for those services. An equally compelling reason for collecting meaningful data, however, is that what clinicians learn from each patient can be enhanced by applying appropriate controls and designs to measure the effects of treatment. Clinically rigorous designs also provide evidence supporting decisions to begin, modify, or terminate treatment.

### The Scientific Method in the Clinic

The five basic components of the scientific method are not much different from treatment as it is generally thought of. These five components are operational definitions, reliability, dependent variables, independent variables, and control.

Forming operational definitions involves defining the concept as an overt, measurable unit. An operational definition of auditory comprehension, for example, might be the response, in a pointing task, to the presentation of single words auditorily.

*Reliability* refers to the likelihood that a particular response will be measured the same way, either by one tester at different times, by more than one tester, or in different situations. The more controls there are for internal validity and the more careful the observer, the greater the reliability. The importance of reliability lies in the necessity of describing a behavior precisely and unvaryingly, so that change can be measured and observed independent of other variables.

*Control* refers to the precision used to regulate the independent variables. These variables may involve timing, frequency, intensity, salience, redundancy, and others that the clinician can vary in the presentation of the independent variable.

Much of the single-case research in the past few years has been descriptive or correlational. That is, behaviors have been observed, and then described or correlated, but with no manipulation of experimental variables. There are two types of experimental variables in clinical research: Dependent variables are the behaviors to be observed and measured; independent or treatment variables are the variables manipulated by the clinician to see if the treatment results in a change in observed behavior (dependent variable).

## Single-Case Designs in the Treatment of Global Aphasia

Because they permit precision and organization in treatment, the most useful and appropriate designs for studying the effects of a treatment on a single patient are single-case, or time-series, designs. (Single-case designs for the treatment of speech and language disorders are handled elegantly, and in much greater depth, by McReynolds and Kearns [1983].) A brief summary of them is presented here because only a few single-case designs are appropriate—under certain conditions—for the globally aphasic patient.

The three major divisions of single-case designs are the within series, the between series, and combined series designs. Within series designs are appropriate for investigating whether the independent variable is responsible for behavior change in a patient. In these designs, a series of measurements are taken successively over time within phases. Between series designs allow comparisons of two or more treatments or conditions in order to examine relative effectiveness on a given outcome measure. Combined series designs combine within and between series strategies.

Selection of the appropriate design for a particular patient is influenced by a number of factors, including anticipated availability for treatment, treatment frequency, rate of recovery, and response to stimulation. Behaviors that are expected to respond rapidly to treatment are probably best assessed with between series designs. Several within series designs and combined series designs are more appropriate for behaviors that are expected to change relatively slowly.

## Withdrawal Designs

Withdrawal designs, a type of within series design, are often thought best suited to evaluate the effects of a reversible procedure. The treatment effect is inferred from the response on a particular task, following baseline testing, over time. If treatment that has been effective is withdrawn, the anticipated response is a decline in performance on that particular task.

A typical withdrawal design begins with a baseline, or A, phase, in which the behavior to be treated is tested. Three consecutive baselines should be collected and, if possible, should be counterbalanced across conditions (e.g., morning, afternoon, afternoon, morning). Once the baseline phase is complete, treatment can be applied. In this, the B phase, treatment may be applied over one or more sessions, but the probes should be as systematic as possible and should be administered at the same time increments. Once criterion has been reached and stabilized for two or three sessions, treatment is typically withdrawn (hence the term withdrawal). If the treatment has been effective, there is a tendency for that behavior to decline slightly, demonstrating the treatment's effect, but there should not be a return to baseline levels.

The major criticism against withdrawal designs is an ethical one: If treatment has been effective, it is unethical to withdraw it. That criticism would be particularly appropriate for administering medications that do not have a lasting effect but produce relief from symptoms only when administered regularly. Treatment for aphasia, on the other hand, is generally thought to have a lasting effect (i.e., relief from symptoms is thought to endure once treatment has ended) and no evidence suggests that withdrawal of treatment deprives a patient of the gains made. Collins and Wertz (1983) found no significant differences between performance on selected speech and language measures administered immediately upon ending intensive treatment and the same measures administered up to several years post onset. To avoid such criticism, many clinicians use withdrawal designs that allow measurement of the effects of withdrawal and the implied effects of treatment, and apply treatment again in a final phase, the B phase. This design, called an

ABAB, is probably the most widely used and the most useful of the single-case designs. A typical ABAB design is shown in Figure 6–1. In this graph the behavior being treated is auditory recognition of single words to be selected from two written foils. The scoring system is the PICA 16 point scale. The graph shows that baseline performance over three sessions is relatively flat. When treatment is applied, in the B phase, performance accelerates and finally stabilizes at approximately 80 percent correct (a correct response in this case is accurate performance after a repetition of the stimulus).

A useful tool for recording and graphing responses is the Base-10 response form (LaPointe, 1977) shown in Figure 6–2. On this form, variables that affect the independent variable, the treatment, can be noted, as can the controls on the dependent variable (e.g., scoring used and criterion for success); and performance on each response can be recorded and summarized with a mean score or percentage.

LaPointe's form (1975) provides an efficient means of summarizing and displaying responses based on Base-10 Programmed stimulation. This

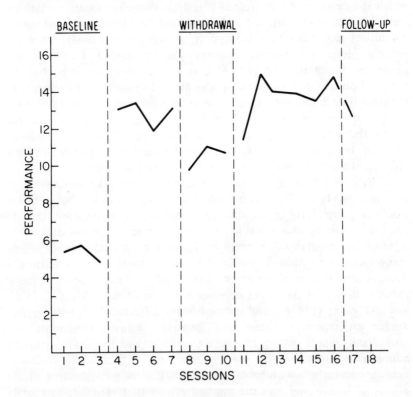

**Figure 6–1.** A typical ABAB design with extended follow-up.

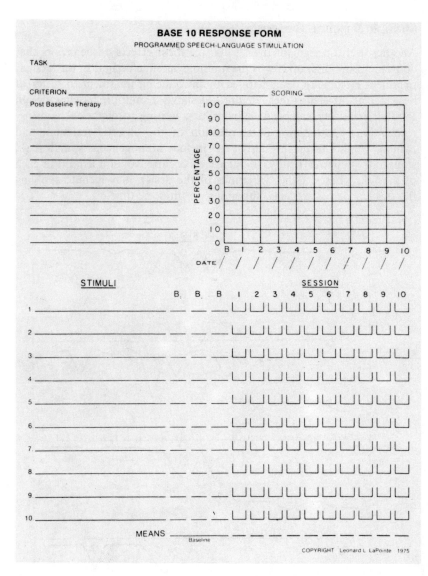

**Figure 6–2.** Base-10 response form for displaying and summarizing responses.

program is really an amalgamation of programmed or operant principles and stimulation-facilitation treatment. These principles include clearly defined tasks; baseline performance measurement; session-by-session progress plotting; and graphic displays of changes in performance.

## Multiple Baseline Designs

Another useful design for measuring treatment effects on behaviors that do not improve dramatically is the multiple baseline design. In this design, treatment effects are demonstrated by introducing treatment to different baselines at different times. Figure 6–3 shows a multiple baseline design for four relatively independent behaviors: writing to dictation, auditory recognition, pantomimed demonstration of the object's function, and naming. Variations on this design can include homogeneous stimuli (e.g., stimuli of similar difficulty, frequency of occurrence, and length) in each of the four phases. Other variations of the design may include applying the strategy across subjects, situations, settings, or time.

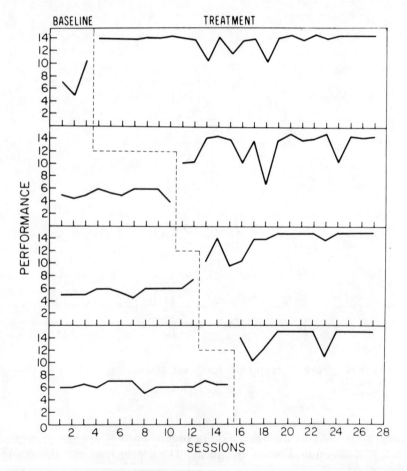

**Figure 6–3.** Typical multiple baseline design for measuring treatment effects on multiple behavioral targets.

Once baselines have been collected, treatment is applied to the first phase, writing to dictation. The probes are administered to all four phases at the same times; the three remaining phases, however, are not treated until criterion has been achieved on the first phase. At that point, treatment is applied to the second phase, and the process continues until all phases have been treated. One variation of the design includes the withdrawal of treatment for the phase just completed, but most clinicians prefer to continue to treat all phases in sequential order.

In this example, performance on writing to dictation had reached criterion—80 percent correct with one repetition—by the sixth treatment session. The modest improvement in the untreated phases suggests either that there was some generalization across phases from the treatment or that an uncontrolled variable (e.g., spontaneous recovery) accounted for the improvement. Generally, in this design the clinician is assured that treatment is effective when a change in responses appears after its application while the level of untreated behavior remains relatively constant. Independence of treatment targets is nearly impossible in speech and language treatment, however, and some improvement in untreated items is not unexpected. Because the differences in performance on the untreated phases are so great compared with the treated phases, the clinician can be relatively certain that performance is influenced by the treatment and not by any other unexplained variable.

## MICROCOMPUTERS IN APHASIA

In reviewing the use of microcomputers in clinical management of the aphasic patient, LaPointe (1984) found that they are being used for

1. Direct word retrieval and communication aids.
2. Adaptation and development of software designed for aphasia treatment.
3. Clinical administration and data retrieval.
4. Prediction, prognosis, estimation of treatment duration, and the plotting of acceleration rates and slopes of performance.

Nevertheless, most microcomputer activity has focused on treatment, and the vast majority of software development for aphasia has focused on the mildly to moderately affected patient. Only one study extant, for example, has investigated the efficacy of microcomputers as an alternative form of communication in global aphasia. Helm-Estabrooks and Walsh (1982) used a word board and microprocessor linked to a monitor (SPLINK) containing 950 commonly used words and phrases, the alphabet, and numbers, and with the capacity to perform a number of linguistic activities. These included spelling words, joining two or more words together to yield a new word, punctuating and capitalizing, correcting errors, and modifying existing words. The researchers employed a 10 step program to train 13 aphasic patients, and then compared their natural communication ability with SPLINK communication.

They found that no patient achieved a higher level of communication than with his or her own spoken, written, or gestural output, and that even globally aphasic patients tended to communicate more using a few words, with intonation changes, facial expressions, and simple gestures, than with SPLINK.

Despite what might be construed as negative results, the future of the microcomputer as augmentative or alternative communication for severely and globally aphasic patients promises to be bright. The power of small, even portable microcomputers is growing at an almost alarming rate (alarming, that is, for those who purchased 32K and 64K machines 2 years ago). Today it is possible to purchase machines with four to eight times that memory at similar cost. For a bit more money, hard or floppy disk drives with 5 to 40 megabyte capacities are readily available, providing memory capacities similar to those of mainframe computers 10 years ago. Laser technology, including storage and retrieval capacities, and such advances as bubble memory are threatening to make even these awesome memories obsolete. Memory may be the most important single factor in the development of smart and functional alternative and augmentative communication devices for aphasic patients. Adapting associational memories, graphic displays, and menus for use by language handicapped individuals requires tremendous amounts of memory. The average microcomputer of today does not approach these memory requirements, but tomorrow's probably will.

Computer-assisted rehabilitation is not only a practical adjunct to traditional face-to-face treatment and evaluation; it may be even more than that. At the present time, three basic options or combinations of options are available to the clinician who would treat global aphasia: treatment, which may be machine- or computer-assisted (e.g., microcomputer, Language Masters); assistive devices employed to enable a patient to communicate through normal channels (e.g., Melodic Intonation); and augmentative, in which a behavior more accessible to the patient is substituted for the more usual form of communication (e.g., a communication board for the speechless patient).

Numerous factors may interact in selecting one of the three options. Patients with mild forms of aphasia and rapid recovery may never require assistive or augmentative forms, or may require them only briefly. The severely afflicted patient may never be able to take advantage of assistive devices and may benefit from more intensive treatment in the use of an augmentative system. Even the most advanced options available, however, have not kept pace with current technology. Why this is so is unclear. It may be that "a patient who can use a sophisticated augmentative or assistive device probably doesn't need it" is a particularly pervasive viewpoint in the management of aphasia. This view, it seems, is shallow, because it imperils innovative techniques and overlooks the residual skills of even the most severely aphasic patients.

As noted earlier, numerous investigators have demonstrated that globally aphasic patients retain significant logical or cognitive capacities. Current technology has the capacity to focus messages by asking nonverbal questions, correcting incorrect inputs, inhibiting perseveration, and escorting the patient through a logical series of choices, which can be displayed verbally, nonverbally, pictorially, or symbolically. This technology and the residual perceptual and cognitive skills possessed by severely aphasic patients adequately support the hypothesis that the two can be yoked to provide much more effective augmentative and assistive systems for the severely aphasic patient.

Several arguments indicate the value of introducing computerized rehabilitative efforts:

1. Devices which operate somewhat independently of the clinician free therapists for other duties. This semi-independent functioning also contributes to the patient's feeling of responsibility and control over his environment and rehabilitation, thereby enhancing the learning process (Katz and Tong-Nagy, 1982).
2. Diagnostic and assessment tasks can be presented and responses recorded without any examiner bias.
3. Computer-assisted rehabilitation provides valuable supplementary language therapy; presently, many aphasic individuals are denied adequate treatment until clinicians are available to treat them.
4. Patients may be able to use equipment during "off-hours" when they are not fatigued.
5. Home-based therapy can be accomplished on portable or remote-control equipment.
6. The routine aspects of aphasia therapy, such as repetitious practice, are highly compatible with machine capabilities (Holland, 1970).
7. Benefit-cost ratios are likely to be high. Significant costs of equipment (which are declining rapidly) are offset by the increased number of patients who receive therapy.

The relatively recent emergence of computer-assisted diagnosis and treatment of speech and language disorders has been succeeded by a formidable rationale for use of computers, in particular extolling their benefits to the patient. Additional advantages that are frequently overlooked are the cost-efficiency of data collection and the precision of computerized administration, scoring, and analysis of evaluation measures. Odell and associates (1985) recently investigated microcomputer-assisted assessment of visual problem-solving ability in global aphasia. They designed a computerized version of Raven's *Coloured Progressive Matrices* (Raven, 1962), a frequently used measure in the diagnosis of aphasia and related disorders. Their version of the test was implemented on an IBM PC with 576K of random access memory (RAM), a Tecmar PC-Mate Graphics color generation board, dual disk drives, a standard keyboard, and a TSD touch-sensitive screen mounted on an Electrochrome RGB color monitor. The input device, the touch-sensitive screen, allowed the patients to simply touch the screen to indicate the correct answer. One additional major modification to the test was the addition of four practice items to familiarize patients with the test and the procedure.

This version of the test permitted both automatic operation and patient control of items presented, self-correction of errors, and an immediate summary of performance on a number of parameters, including reaction time for each item, total reaction time, total time required for the test, percentiles for normal and brain-damaged subjects, and analysis of error type and problem type. The test is well standardized and reliable and correlates highly with the traditional version.

Odell and associates administered this test to five globally aphasic patients. All patients were tested at least one month following a single left hemisphere CVA, all had right hemiplegia, and none had peripheral sensory losses which prevented their participation. Overall communicative ability as measured by the PICA ranged between the 10th and 25th percentiles for aphasic adults.

The researchers found that, despite the severity of the patients' linguistic and cognitive impairment, none required more than the four practice trials and minimal clinician assistance to learn the task in either condition. Total scores ranged from 4 to 29 for condition A (computer-controlled) to 3 to 29 for condition B (rate of presentation controlled by the patient). The scores for both conditions are compatible with the patients' performance on the standard version of the test.

Error types and problem types were similar across patients, with errors of type C predominating (repetition of the pattern).

The results suggest that computerized assessment in global aphasia is not only possible but useful and expeditious. In this particular version of the test, ease of interaction between machine and patient is facilitated, to the patients' benefit, and the clinician is rewarded by the precision, speed, and power of computer-assisted assessment in aphasia.

## Computerized Treatment in Global Aphasia

In addition to the human cost incurred by the devastating impact of global aphasia, the indirect costs (including loss of earning power, rehabilitation support, and ancillary services) approach $4 billion annually in the United States alone. That figure does not include salaries for speech clinicians. Computerized treatment devices have the potential to increase substantially the number of patients seen for evaluation and treatment, reduce the number of patients awaiting treatment, and significantly reduce the per-visit cost. A recent study at the Birmingham, Alabama, Veterans Administration Hospital estimated the per-visit cost for traditional visits in the United States at $48.62. Through use of the locally developed REMATE system, which provides therapy from a hospital computer to veterans in their own homes, staff time and cost per visit have been reduced tremendously—in some cases (e.g., telephone interface with a central computer) to $1.33. More important, perhaps, are the significant increase in number of patients treated through computer-assisted programs, and the potential of even greater impact from such projects in the near future.

Many of these projects use relatively inexpensive microcomputers such as the Apple II or the IBM PC. These devices are adequate for most purposes. Because of the large amount of textual data involved in language therapy, however, a key component of such systems will be a so-called "hard" disk, which can network single task systems into a common data base and can also store 5 to 40 million characters of information. One benefit of using this new technology instead of floppy disks is the elimination of time-consuming searching and swapping during therapy sessions.

Recent advances have resulted in the increasingly successful application of computer technology both to the rehabilitation of patients with a variety of communication disorders and to the investigation of brain mechanisms underlying aphasia. This advanced technology, however, is inadequately used for the severely aphasic patient.

The value of introducing electromechanical, electronic, and computerized devices into a traditionally interpersonal rehabilitation process is therefore supported by several arguments: (1) such equipment is intended not to replace conventional face-to-face therapy but rather to complement it; (2) devices that operate somewhat independently of the clinician free therapists for other duties; (3) this semi-independent functioning also gives patients a feeling of responsibility and control over the environment and the therapy, thereby enhancing the rehabilitation process; (4) patients may be able to use equipment during "off" hours to continue therapy when they are not fatigued; (5) home-based therapy can be accomplished on portable or remote-control equipment; (6) routine aspects of aphasia therapy, such as repetitious practice, are highly compatible with machine capabilities; (7) benefit-cost ratios are likely to be high: significant initial costs of equipment are offset by the increased number of patients who receive therapy; (8) computer-assisted, alternative communication devices are now technologically feasible.

Although a fairly substantial body of literature exists that demonstrates the successful application of microcomputer-based systems to the treatment of aphasia, the microcomputer is rarely employed as an augmentative or alternative communication device. Recently, however, several computerized devices have been developed as "language prostheses"; these units aid aphasic individuals in retrieving linguistic information, organizing it into acceptable linguistic structures, and enhancing their own restricted output. Colby and colleagues (1981) programmed a portable microprocessor to assist anomic aphasic people in finding specific words in conversation. The computer cues the user by requesting precise information about the desired word, such as topic area, an associated word, and first, middle, or last letter. Pertinent vocabulary is programmed for later production by the voice synthesizer, but the lexicon is flexible; seldom-used words are automatically deleted, while the user can add new items.

A program that dramatically enhances and elaborates on a user-supplied message has been developed by Hillinger and associates (1981). In this program syntactically incomplete language input is transformed into complete, grammatical utterances. The input is elaborated in two ways: by encoding principles, in which a single word (e.g., "bathroom") actually represents and activates multiple words (e.g., "I need to go to the bathroom"); and by computer processing, in which user commands concerning syntactical options, such as "past" or "negative," are manipulated into grammatical utterances by transformational rules in the software.

These aids are designed for adults with mild or moderate language impairment who are able to read and spell at least in some elementary fashion. Little attention, however, has been paid to the communication needs of severely or globally aphasic patients.

If, as noted earlier, the "primary pathways" that remain intact in global aphasia are the ones that do not require verbal mediation, a logical channel of communication is at least suggested: pictorial representation of verbal messages. Because the concepts that can be expressed with communication boards are inadequate for most forms of communication, "smart" microprocessors that can anticipate requests with only minimal cues can focus messages by asking nonverbal questions, correcting incorrect inputs, and escorting the individual through a logical series of choices displayed verbally or nonverbally. This technology, using the residual perceptual and cognitive skills possessed by severely aphasic individuals, suggests that much more effective augmentative and alternative communication systems for globally aphasic individual can be developed using available microcomputers, software, and keyboard emulators. Preliminary testing of available treatment programs with globally aphasic patients suggestd that the computer might be uniquely suited to enhancing the residual capabilities of the globally aphasic patient and might provide the kind of repetition and feedback required by these patients. In the author's clinic, we have begun treating globally aphasic patients with programs designed to improve spelling and reading comprehension.

At present most projects remain in the conceptual stages. One preliminary project, however, was recently begun by Collins and Odell. They plan to test the efficacy of four input devices: the traditional typewriter-based keyboard (keyboard emulator), long and short range light pens, a touch-sensitive screen, and a joy stick.

Two of the more significant hindrances to microcomputer use in global aphasia are self-correction and perseveration. Self-correction occurs when the individual produces a response, scans it visually or auditorily, and makes appropriate adjustments in his or her output. Allowing for self-correction is relatively easy provided that sufficient time is given and that the individual retains adequate recognition of the target and is aided by appropriate linguistic or extra-linguistic cues. Tolerable limits for these parameters vary somewhat but high-speed information exchange is the norm, and although normal communicators employ self-correction, they require little time to implement it. Aphasic patients whose retrieval mechanisms operate inefficiently require a great deal more time.

Perseveration is the failure to discontinue a response once it is no longer appropriate. It is a maladaptive response that is difficult to control even by the clinician's active intervention. Its mechanisms are not well understood, but several hypotheses exist. Muma and McNeil (1981) suggested that perseveration may be the result of hypofunctioning of the "volitional mechanism" (p. 214) and noted that the problem is common in aphasia. Porch (1981) suggested that the problem is pervasive even when the task is not difficult and the patient is not overly tired and is emotionally stable. In the author's experience, perseveration is most frequently encountered in the acute stage but persists in most patients throughout the recovery period, although the frequency drops with recovery and the behavior is easier to overcome. As Sparks (1981) suggested, the inherent danger is not controlling perseveration is that perseverative repetitions of an error reinforce that inappropriate response.

It is clear that perseveration constitutes a significant hindrance to functional communication. What is not clear, however, is whether it results from a failure to recognize the inappropriate response or from an inability to alter the response once it is established. There is no consensus on the most effective means of disrupting the perseverative response. Rosenberg and Edwards (1965) found that perseverative tendencies were disrupted by the sounding of a loud buzzer as "punishment." Others (Muma and McNeil, 1981) limited intervention to several brief periods or provided a number of different tasks and response requirements (Porch, 1981).

Any computer-assisted program in which the patient is required to work independently must recognize perseveration and alter the patient's behavior accordingly. A suitable program for severely or globally aphasic patients, then, should allow the patient himself to modify the response (self-correct), or should insert some alerting device, to (1) prevent "learning" of maladaptive responses; (2) identify appropriate measures to prevent perseveration for both computer-assisted and face-to-face treatment; (3) enhance efficiency of communication; and (4) reduce frustration and fatigue in treatment tasks.

At this time, computer-assisted treatment programs that have been developed do not address the issues of computer recognition of perseveration or facilitation of self-correction attempts. An auditory comprehension program designed by Mills (1982) does enable the individual to request a repeat of the stimulus item, but there is no mechanism to correct a response already entered into the computer. More recent programs seem more sensitive to self-correction and perseveration.

Several programs proven useful in the rehabilitation of global aphasia are discussed in Chapter 8. These programs capitalize mostly on the display characteristics of basic microcomputers, and they do not require sophisticated graphics capabilities or highly audible digitized or synthesized voice. Most require at least minimal reading recognition skills and only minimal facility with a keyboard to input responses. The majority of globally aphasic patients have little difficulty learning to use a full keyboard. In some cases clinicians have isolated certain needed keys or marked the keys required for a particular program with colored tape.

The complaint most often heard from aphasia clinicians is that there is not much usable software available for aphasia treatment. It is true that there is little available commercially, but a number of public domain or user-designed programs are available. An excellent source for those programs is a group called Computer Users in Speech and Hearing (CUSH) at Ohio University. This group is compiling a software registry for diagnosis, treatment, patient data management, and clinical teaching in speech, language, and hearing. Another excellent source for inexpensive, copyable programs is the local users' group for the different computer manufacturers.

## MAINTENANCE TREATMENT

Barring new illnesses, years of aging, or drastic changes in environment aphasic patients maintain the gains they have made once they have left treatment. Most, in fact, get better. Should clinicians continue to treat patients once they have achieved optimal treatment benefits and, if so, with what frequency and toward what goal?

The answer lies in the patient. Those who aspire to improve communication skills or who willingly accept their family's aspirations should probably be treated, provided that clinicians can justify the treatment with even minimal gains in communicative skills. Others are more reluctant to continue traditional or group treatment beyond a more or less arbitrary time frame. West (in Aten et al., 1981) said that "the sooner a patient is discharged from all therapies the quicker his adjustment to what is his particular reality" (p. 150). West advocates intensive treatment for an inpatient—frequently with group therapy as an adjunct—until discharge or the point at which the patient has received maximal hospital benefit. Then the patient enters a Discharge Planning group which focuses on practical issues in daily living and adjustment. While the patient is in this group, the family participates simultaneously in a separate group with a similar focus. After discharge, the patient joins a community involvement group that emphasizes the development and acceptance of alternative life styles, stressing activities the patient can do rather than what he or she cannot do. Patients typically attend this group for 4 to 8 months. After that time, they attend only the stroke club. West believes that "continuing to come to the hospital focuses on what the patient cannot do and becomes ultimately counter-productive to good rehabilitation" (p. 150), and that "as long as a patient is still receiving occupational or physical therapy, treatment from speech pathology, or the like, he tends not to come to grips with what his disability is and will continue to be" (p. 150).

West's view has merit, but not all clinicians share the assurance that continued treatment is unwarranted, nor is there any evidence that those patients would not continue to make gains. Broida (1977) among others found that even chronically aphasic patients make significant gains when treated.

Maintenance therapy (i.e., traditional, one-to-one client-clinician relationships) for the sale of maintaining skills previously acquired is probably unjustified. If skills erode, then a second, or even a third, period of intensive treatment is justified. If particular needs emerge because of a change in life style, reconsultation and application of treatment are probably justified. It is much easier to justify group treatment.

## TERMINATING TREATMENT

Criteria for terminating treatment vary widely. The general consensus, however, seems to be that treatment of severely aphasic patients should be discontinued when they (1) have received appropriate speech and language treatment on an optimal schedule; (2) fail to achieve treatment goals; (3) fail to show significant progress (poor scores) on reassessment batteries and functional measures; (4) fail to exhibit significant change following a 2 month treatment period.

Formal tests, even of "functional" abilities, may not accurately reflect a patient's improvement, and artificially contrived situations may not elicit the competence the clinician has tried to train. The truest test may be covert observation in natural settings. Some clinicians (Holland, 1982, for example) are fortunate enough to be observers "in vivo," but find the collection of data repugnant or obtrusive. It is also expensive. Systematic questionnaires of the type discussed earlier may be the best compromise. If obtained by an observant caregiver, not only do they tell us what patients can do and whether they are successful at tasks worked on, but also such questionnaires help clinicians address the functional communication needs of patients in treatment.

Most patients will save clinicians the trouble of deciding an appropriate time to terminate treatment. They begin to come in less frequently, or ask to be seen less frequently, or call to say that their car is permanently broken. That should be a hint. Generally, the patients are saying one of several things: (1) treatment no longer holds the promise of success; (2) the importance of communication has become secondary to spending time with friends and family; (3) treatment has become a financial or emotional burden that can no longer be endured; (4) they have reached an acceptable level of communicative independence, and by compromising can get on with their lives.

Speech pathologists need not feel they have not done an adequate job when patients decide to terminate treatment. In some way, they have helped each patient to make a very serious and thoughtful decision. Clinicians should wish them well, give them a business card, and accept the situation.

More difficult for the clinician is deciding when to terminate treatment for a patient who is unwilling or unable to make that decision independently. Concern for the patient, moral obligation, and (possibly) equally compelling desires to be both objective and realistic make it difficult to determine when treatment—not *a* treatment—has ceased to be effective or when potential gains do not justify the cost. Warren (1976), summarizing a panel discussion, says that the decision to terminate is based on the clinician's prediction of the effectiveness of continued treatment, treatment logistics, and the clinician's concern about the patient, and should include the interaction of patient characteristics, test and treatment data, treatment goals, clinical and financial arrangements, system pressures, and the ethical and moral viewpoints of the clinician.

Theoretically, it might be possible to assign weights to each factor and create an equation to tell us when to terminate treatment. Termination usually becomes an issue when a patient fails to make clinically or statistically significant progress on treated tasks. As if the patient were a contestant in some vaguely dangerous educational game, the "judges" are the clinician, the spouse, the physician, the bursar, and (frequently) the calendar.

The easiest termination decision, but probably the most emotionally bruising, is the one enforced by family finances. Few clinicians are philanthropists, although most might like to be, and once the patient's financial lifeline is cut, treatment cannot be continued unless supplemental funding is found.

## SUMMARY

The treatments discussed in Chapters 5 and 6 have highlighted some general and specific considerations applicable to many aphasic patients. The majority are appropriate solely for globally aphasic patients. If there are other considerations, they are anecdotal or unpublished. These general considerations will serve as guidelines in the management of globally aphasic patients.

Chapters 7 and 8 present specific procedures for the treatment of global aphasia and demonstrate their application to three patients with very different varieties of global aphasia. In another form, these procedures might be appropriate for patients who, in the early stages of recovery, are expected to make significant gains in communication; more appropriate procedures for these patients, however, probably include approaches such as stimulation (Duffy, 1981), divergent semantic intervention (Chapey, 1981), or other approaches particularly suited to those patients' needs—that is, treatment for apraxia of speech, intersystemic reorganization, or melodic intonation therapy.

The treatments discussed in Chapters 7 and 8 are designed to be implemented with severe, relatively unremitting global aphasia. Signs that the condition is evolving should prompt another avenue of intervention.

# Appendix 6–1

## SUGGESTED READINGS FOR THE FAMILIES OF GLOBALLY APHASIC PATIENTS

*About stroke* (1978). Minneapolis: Sister Kenny Institute, Rehabilitation Publication 724.

American Heart Association, 7320 Greenville Ave., Dallas, TX: 75231.

American Heart Association. *Stroke: A guide for the family.* Dallas, TX: American Heart Association.

Boone, D.R. (1965). *An adult has aphasia.* Danville, IL: The Interstate Printers and Publishers, Inc.

Broida, H. (1979). *Coping with stroke.* San Diego: College-Hill Press.

Brubaker, S.H. (1982). *Sourcebook for aphasia: A guide to family activities and community resources.* Detroit: Wayne State University Press.

Cohen, L.K. (1978). *Communication problems after a stroke.* Minneapolis: Sister Kenny Institute.

Fowler, R.S., and Fordyce, W.E. (1978). *Stroke: Why do they behave that way?* Dallas: American Heart Association, Office of Communication.

McBride, C. (1969). *Silent victory.* Chicago: Nelson-Hall Company.

Sanders, S.B., and Hamby, E.I. (1984). *You are not alone.* Nashville: American Heart Association, Tennessee affiliate.

Sarno, M.T. (1963). *Understanding aphasia: A guide for family and friends.* New York: The Institute of Rehabilitation Medicine, New York University Medical Center.

Serbin, S.J., and Sommers, R.K. (1985). *Aphasia and associated problems.* Kent, OH: Kent State University.

Wolf, H.H. (1979). *Aphasia, my world alone.* Detroit: Wayne State University Press.

# Chapter 7

# Specific Treatments for Global Aphasia

The treatment procedures that follow have been used with some success, and some failure, in this and other clinics. Not all are advocated as efficacious with every globally aphasic person, but all appear worthy of consideration for the clinical armamentarium. With appropriate patients, each technique or combination of techniques may stand alone. Frequently, time imposes limits on treatment that require them to be used exclusively. The ultimate goal of each technique, however, is an incorporation of skills, a fusing of functional communication in the modality (or combination of modalities) that is most appropriate to the individual patient. Functional communication is seen as the result of a pragmatic approach to treatment that capitalizes on and enhances residual skills and focuses on persuading the patient and his or her significant others that communication, not linguistic elegance, is paramount.

Not all of the treatment programs that follow have been designed specifically for the globally aphasic patient. What distinguishes them from many other programs, however, is either a flexibility that permits their effective use with severely (or less severely) involved patients or their recognition that globally aphasic patients require specific techniques that are not appropriate for the more mildly affected patient. This is true of both the general and the more specific programs.

## VISUAL ACTION THERAPY (VAT)

In 1978, Helm and Benson presented the results of a treatment program for global aphasia called Visual Action Therapy. In this program, the patient is trained to associate ideographic forms with particular objects and actions and to carry out a series of tasks in association with these drawings. The rationale for this particular program is based on Helm and Benson's observation that globally aphasic patients were unable to produce meaningful gestures in association with drawings; they thought that the patients might benefit from training in the appreciation and production of symbolic gestures as a precursor to language communication treatment. There were two unique features of this program as it was presented in 1978. First, no verbalization was used during the training, and second, the program was designed to serve as a precursor to language training.

Helm-Estabrooks, Fitzpatrick, and Barresi (1982) have published the only report of the efficacy of this program. Their rationale, method, subjects, results, and discussion are described in some detail here because they are striking, and the application of the program is of significant potential benefit to a large number of patients with severe deficits. They report a significant positive effect from their treatment program. Additional reports of its efficacy have not yet been published, although the program is often extolled anecdotally by clinicians. The authors begin by citing the literature, suggesting that severe deficits in traditional communicative modalities (speaking, writing, reading, auditory comprehension) do not typically yield to traditional therapeutic measures. They present several theoretical rationales to support the training of gestural output systems of global patients: (1) Gestural communication may be used independently of vocal communication; (2) hand gestures for manual communication require less refined motor control than the articulatory movements required for speech communication; (3) limb movements, unlike facial movements, have more predominantly unilateral control. The left arm and hand are innervated by right hemisphere pyramidal pathways, which are presumably uncompromised in right hemiplegic global patients having exclusively left hemisphere lesions; (4) the hand and arm, unlike the bucco-facial apparatus necessary for speech, is visible to the initiator and can be visually monitored.

Despite these theoretical advantages to gestural training, however, Helm-Estabrooks and colleagues (1982) point out that globally aphasic patients may well have severe limb apraxia of the nonhemiplegic left arm, which must be overcome if they are to learn a gestural system, and that severe auditory and reading comprehension disturbances may preclude the use of verbal or written instructions. This can be overcome either by using nonorthographic visual stimuli as a symbol system or by capitalizing on relatively better ability to respond to pantomimed instructions than to verbal instructions for the same tasks.

To test their hypotheses, Helm-Estabrooks and associates (1982) used VAT to treat eight globally aphasic patients who had not responded to traditional therapeutic intervention. All patients were right-handed, right hemiplegic men who ranged in age from 37 to 70 years, and were from 12 to 144 weeks post onset. Their diagnoses were based on severity ratings on the BDAE below 1, overall auditory comprehension score no higher than −1.25, and an absence of naming, repetition, reading, and writing skills. Overall scores on the PICA ranged from 5.61 to 8.22, all of which were below the 25th percentile. Patients were treated in half-hour sessions for approximately five sessions per week and required from 4 to 14 weeks to complete the program.

The program is thoughtfully planned and is laid out in a series of steps that appear to approximate a hierarchy. It is a three level program that uses eight unimanual objects, each of which can be represented with a distinct gesture, and large, realistic colored drawings of each object. The objects are outlined in black and reproduced on 5 × 8 inch index cards, with smaller drawings of each object on 1½ × 3 inch cards, and eight drawings on 3 × 5 inch cards depicting a figure appropriately manipulating each object.

All directions, reinforcements, and procedural steps are nonvocal. The program follows a hierarchy of difficulty, requiring nearly 100 percent success for each step before progressing to the next step. It is advisable to review previous or easier steps at the beginning of each session.

The materials used are eight objects (razor, telephone, cup, toy pistol, saw, hammer, screwdriver, and blackboard eraser) and their contextual prompts if indicated (block of wood, block of wood with protruding nail, block of wood with protruding screw, a slate), large colored line drawings, small colored line drawings of these objects, and drawings depicting the objects being manipulated by a stick figure.

Step 1, Level I of this program is designed to help the patient understand that line drawings of objects can represent real objects, and it is concerned primarily with tracing of the patient's hand, tracing objects, and matching objects to pictures. In Step 2, the patient is required to match objects to pictures and pictures to objects. In Step 3, the patient uses the eight objects and the small object cards to match pictures to objects and objects to pictures. In Step 4, the clinician first demonstrates the function of each object and then asks (nonverbally) the patient to pick up the object and demonstrate its function. The authors say that if the patient has persistent difficulty in manipulating a particular object, it should be removed from the array and a permanent substitute (e.g., a paintbrush) selected. The remaining eight steps allow for "action picture command" instructions, following action picture commands, pantomimed gesture demonstration, recognizing pantomimed gestures, pantomimed gesture instruction, producing pantomimed gestures, pantomimed gesture for absent object demonstration, and producing pantomimed gestures for absent objects. In the two succeeding levels, steps 7 to 12 of the first two levels are repeated, first substituting the action picture cards for the objects, then substituting the small object picture cards for the objects.

When all training was completed, Helm-Estabrooks and colleagues (1982) grouped pretreatment and posttreatment PICA scores for ten subtests: two pantomime tasks and two auditory comprehension tasks, which they labeled Group I and predicted would improve; two reading subtests (Group II), which they predicted might improve; and four verbal subtests (Group III), which they predicted would not improve.

Their predictions were confirmed. Analysis of variance found significant pretreatment and posttreatment effects for Group I, with a significantly larger effect for the gestural subtests than for the auditory subtests, and no significant effects for Groups II and III.

As Helm-Estabrooks and colleagues (1982) present this program, its primary purpose is to train globally aphasic patients to produce representational gestures for visually absent stimuli through the manipulation of real objects. In essence, it is a gestural training program. The unexpected, additional benefits found by the authors are difficult to explain and threaten to diffuse the focus of the program. Studies attempting to validate the results of Helm-Estabrooks and colleagues are under way (DeYoung and McNeil, personal communication, 1985), but published results replicating their findings are unavailable.

Helm-Estabrooks and associates (1982) offer several hypotheses to explain their findings:

1. Patients may employ internal verbal monitoring during the training program.
2. VAT may improve general attentional skills.
3. VAT may improve visual spatial and visual search skills.
4. VAT may reintegrate some of the conceptual systems necessary for linguistic performance.

## ARTIFICIAL LANGUAGE TRAINING

Glass, Gazzaniga, and Premack (1973) modified a system originally developed by Premack (1971) for chimpanzees, in which the primary elements are symbols of varying colors and sizes that are functionally equivalent to words. They used this system to train seven globally aphasic patients on tasks ranging in difficulty from "same-different" to expression and comprehension of simple declarative sentences. Two of the patients progressed to this level of difficulty, and the authors believed that the other patients could have progressed to this level if training had continued. Glass and colleagues conclude that "aphasia may impair symbolization but even in global aphasia the capacity for using symbols is not totally abolished" (p. 102). They surmised that the basic cognitive mechanisms that underlie language might be shared by both hemispheres.

## Novel Pictorial Stimuli

Holland (1977) was "surprised to find no work on teaching aphasics Blissymbols. The Bliss symbol system . . . appears to me to offer significant possibility for the severely impaired aphasic" (p. 10).

## Blissymbols

Blissymbols are pictographs used to represent nouns, verbs, functors, adjectives, and composite words. They are said to be easily intelligible for nonaphasic communication partners, contain a lexicon large enough to allow for the specific needs of the patient in his or her environment, allow for some syntactic structuring, and are handy enough to be carried around and used by a right-sided hemiplegic patient (Archer, 1977). Representative samples of Blissymbols appear in Figure 7-1.

There are several things to consider when contemplating this treatment with globally aphasic adults. First, it should be remembered that apes, regardless of their ontogenetic proximity to humans, possess two intact hemispheres; they are capable of learning relatively complex tasks. They have no experience with language as we know it, and their rewards for learning this "language" are elementary, immediate, and basic. Aphasic individuals, on the other hand, do not possess two intact hemispheres—or even one hemisphere that has been demonstrated unequivocally to possess competence for language. Their experience with language is not nonverbal; their language experience permits them to have memories of using language at or near the highest levels of usage, and the rewards for this competence were frequently subtle and may not have been shared by others. These patients' language allowed them to reason, to postulate, to ponder, to villify, to soothe, and to gain the more subtle rewards of affection and satisfaction. Nonverbal symbols would not seem to satisfy many of the patient's needs, yet clinicians and investigators persist in exploring their effectiveness. Such endeavors are not

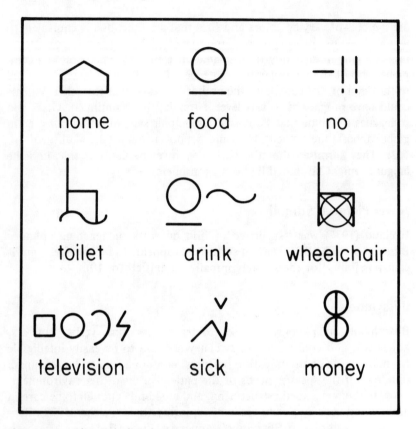

**Figure 7–1.** Blissymbolics for representative words.

folly. The effectiveness of nonverbal symbols with globally aphasic patients who are incapable of learning their linguistic equivalents has not been demonstrated, but they also have not been demonstrated to be ineffective.

A number of reports have found nonverbal symbols to be efficacious with aphasic patients (Bailey, 1978; Kirby, 1978; Lane and Samples, 1981; Saya, 1978).

Horner and LaPointe (1979) evaluated the ability of a severely aphasic patient to learn novel pictorial stimuli (Blissymbols). Their rationale for using novel pictorial stimuli was that (1) they believed the visual and nonphonetic characteristics of the stimuli seemed to lend themselves to right hemisphere processing; (2) "Research findings support the existence of auxiliary right hemisphere mechanisms for processing novel or unfamiliar stimuli"; (3) the clinician can provide the patient with the opportunity for new learning; (4) these stimuli minimize memory load because of the inherent static character of visual stimuli; (5) the task modifies impulsivity and concomitant noise build-up through increased visual scanning and analysis time; (6) the task increases the opportunity for the patient to respond independently of the clinician's auditory-visual cues; (7) the task increases data control because responses to novel stimuli are free of the effects of previous learning.

Through a structured program involving alternating verbal and gestural cues, Horner and LaPointe (1979) tried to determine whether their patient could learn to use available vocabulary for functional communication and what his optimal conditions for learning were. Over 14 days, in 28 sessions, and in 2520 attempts (spontaneous verbalization and elicited verbalization), their patient produced 54 correct utterances spontaneously. His best performance occurred on the second and eighth days, and, both times, his performance subsequently dropped below one correct response per session. Horner and LaPointe concluded that carryover to consistent and functionally appropriate usage at home was virtually nil, but they suggested that perhaps their approach could be used for cost-effective treatment planning by evaluating the patient's ability to learn.

More recently, Johannsen-Horbach, Cegla, Mager, Schempp, and Wallesch (1985) used Blissymbols to treat four patients with chronic global aphasia. In this program, all patients received individual treatment at least twice a week for at least 2 months, with these objectives:

1. The patient should acquire a basic lexicon of nouns, verbs, adjectives, adverbs, and function words, which were chosen according to the patient's individual needs.
2. The patient should learn to produce and understand simple sentences in the symbol language.
3. The patient's relatives should be acquainted with the symbol system so that they could use the symbols in their communication with the patient.

The symbols were introduced to the patient verbally and by simultaneous presentation of pictures or objects or by pantomime by the therapist. The patient first had to associate symbols and pictures in multiple-choice arrays. When this task was performed without errors in 10 trials in two consecutive sessions for five to eight nouns, the first two verbs were introduced in a similar way. Function words were demonstrated by thematic pictures. As soon as possible, Blissymbol sentences were used in therapy and question pronouns were introduced, so that therapeutic communication could be based on symbols. Proficiency of communication was assessed by using correct answers to questions posed in Blissymbolics concerning thematic pictures as a parameter of the symbol lexicon and the use of symbols in the communication at home as an indicator of benefit from therapy.

The results of the treatment by Johannsen-Horbach and colleagues (1985) were mixed but persuasive. They found that despite the failure of these patients to benefit from conventional language rehabilitation programs, all patients acquired a symbol lexicon, and all patients even understood the meaning of function word symbols. Three of the four patients could produce syntactically correct sentences (in Blissymbols) in response to thematic pictures of questions in Blissymbols. Two of the patients used the symbols in their communication with their relatives, and one used phrases. An astonishing finding is that three of the four patients began to articulate the correct word simultaneously while pointing to the correct word, and one patient even articulated simultaneously grammatical sentences in response to questions in Blissymbols. Johannsen-Horbach and colleagues surmise that this could support the theory of Weigl and Bierwisch (1970) that language competence remains largely undisturbed by aphasia, but they prefer the explanation that

> the grammatically correct form is the most probable realization of the lexical content of a statement. Simple sentences such as those articulated simultaneously have premorbidly been called up only in a grammatical form. We assume a phonemic-motor store which includes stereotyped phrases, highly overlearned sequences, and frequently occurring flection morphemes. This store should of course be subordinated to the generator of the lexical content, but there should also be a nonsemantic access, which is reflected in the intact production of highly overlearned sequences in some global aphasics and in the flection of echolalic responses. This access is possibly also activated with the mediation of the symbol language. (pp. 81–82)

Johannsen-Horback and associates (1985) end on a less optimistic note:

> The question remains whether Blissymbols can be used as the sole means of language rehabilitation in severe aphasics. The one patient in our study who had almost no language production under any condition, including repetition, showed very limited improvement with the symbols. (p. 82)

## PROMOTING APHASICS' COMMUNICATIVE EFFECTIVENESS (PACE)

One of the most elegant and perceptive programs for enhancing communication in the aphasic patient was developed by Davis and Wilcox (1985). Although not specifically designed for use with globally aphasic patients, the PACE program is appropriate for them as well because it emphasizes natural conversational interaction rather than linguistic accuracy. In addition, it recognizes that although not all communicative channels are open to globally aphasic persons, these people may succeed when given free choice of responses even if the choice includes several response modes simultaneously or successively. The program is based on four basic principles: (1) the clinician and patient participate equally as senders and receivers of messages; (2) there is an exchange of new information between the clinician and the patient; (3) the patient has a free choice as to which communicative channels (modalities) he or she will use to convey new information; and (4) feedback is provided by the clinician, as a receiver, in response to the patient's success in conveying a message. The emphasis is not on communicative "accuracy" but on effectively conveying messages, and Davis (1982) reported that a small number of severely impaired patients have been able to communicate on a limited basis within the structure of PACE by using nonverbal channels.

## TREATING EXPRESSIVE ABILITIES

### Treating the Equivocal Response

Globally aphasic patients can understand more than they can express. Although some messages might not be confusing to them, their "yes" and "no" responses often are equivocal and present a more significant barrier to communication than impaired comprehension. Establishing an unequivocal "yes" and "no" repertoire is essential because it establishes a communicative lifeline that can be broken only by hurried questions and impatient listeners. Responses can be verbal or gestural, but it is more important that the responses are clear and unequivocal.

An outline of a typical program for shaping and stabilizing the response is outlined here. In this program, the focus is on getting clear signals in and clear signals out.

1.  Shaping the Response
    a.  First, make it very clear to the patient what is required of him or her. You might begin by saying "We need to work on 'yes' and 'no.' I'm going to say the word, and I want you to watch and listen while I say 'yes' (plus gesture) [pause], and 'no' (plus gesture)." Begin with two 3 × 5 inch cards, with "yes" printed on one and "no" printed on the other. Present either card. Point to the card and very clearly say the word accompanied by the appropriate gesture. Pause 5 seconds, then repeat the word and gesture. Repeat five times in succession. Repeat the procedure for the opposite response.
    b.  Physically assist the patient with five repetitions of "yes" (head nod).
    c.  Physically assist the patient with five repetitions of "no" (side to side head movements) while the clinician says "no."

    d.  Alternate four, then three, then two "yes" and "no" with phys-
ical assistance while clinician says the word. Pause approximately 5 seconds between responses. Responses must always be
corrected.

    e.  Request gestured "no" responses to two simple unambiguous
questions while the clinician assists with gestures and says the
word. Work on these until responses are stabilized.

    f.  Request five repetitions of gestured "yes," then "no." Facilitate
with physical or verbal cues if necessary.

    g.  Request alternating "yes," then "no," at approximately 5 sec-
ond intervals, facilitating the response if required.

2.  Stabilizing the Response

    a.  Request gestured response to simple questions, facilitating if
required.

    b.  Permit only "yes" or "no" response (verbal or gestural) while
playing "21."

    c.  Baseline, then begin treatment of personal, environmental, and
informational questions.

## Gestural Communication

Gestural reorganization has been suggested as treatment for severely
apractic patients (Rosenbek, Collins, and Wertz, 1976; Skelly, Schinsky,
Smith, and Fust, 1974), and gestural language has been suggested as an
alternative mode of communication for a variety of aphasic patients.
The evidence is that gestural, symbolic comprehension and expression
are impaired in aphasia, and particularly in global aphasia, but globally
aphasic patients may benefit from pantomimed instruction and combined pantomime and verbal instructions. Anecdotal support for this is
abundant. It comes from nursing staff, who report that severely aphasic
patients understand everything because they follow pantomimed instructions (or spoken and inadvertently pantomimed instructions). Those
who deal frequently with patients with comprehension deficits find
themselves adopting strategies, perhaps unconsciously, that enable them
to deal more effectively with these patients.

    The author's program for gestural communication is both prag-
matic and exploitative. We probe to discover relatively intact abilities or
those that appear responsive to treatment. We begin by assessing spontaneous gestural ability informally in conversation; formally in response to
pictured or auditory stimuli; and imitatively. Any gestures produced,
even if they do not convey a complete concept, are noted and serve as a
limited core to expand on. A part of each session is devoted to training
in these gestures. If they do not yield to treatment, or if only one or a

few do, gestural treatment is deemphasized for those gestures which did not improve and treatment for them is put in a maintenance phase. The recalcitrant gestures are periodically tested, and if any appear to be yielding they are added to the treatment core. Real objects are used when pantomime fails.

Pointing should be an integral part of any gestural program. When used alone, pointing conveys a message succinctly. When accompanied by verbal or nonverbal facilitators, such as facial expression, speech, or writing, it illuminates the message. Pointing, as an integral part of total communication, can be used to impart a primary message and to convey attributes of an object or concept. The first step in incorporating contextual pointing in a program of total communication is to establish a clear, unequivocal gesture.

The pointing response is not one that requires extensive drill. Most patients use the gesture spontaneously, although their targets may be inappropriate or ambiguous. What they may fail to realize, and may need to be taught, is the power of pointing. Treatment should concentrate on what is pointed to, and its power to communicate, rather than what is used to point with.

A general outline for this gestural program is shown in Table 7-1. One gesture is chosen and is presented in both spoken and gestured form. This gesture is drilled until it is intact, then expanded to two gestures. When that level is reached, the clinician alternates between the two, with fewer repetitions of each until the patient can alternate gestures successively through the final step. At this point, a third gesture is added and the process repeated until all three gestures are firmly established. Additional gestures are added in this way as competence is demonstrated.

Once the patient has learned several gestures, uses them in response to questions, and recognizes the need for them, they are incorporated into a program of total communication, as is discussed later.

## Treating Writing

Writing will probably never be a functional, independent expressive modality for a globally aphasic patient, but even an approximation of a verb or a noun can be persuasive. Part of each treatment session should be devoted to writing drill. Stimuli should be meaningful and salient. The patient's name and family names are often least resistant to treatment, and provide a good place to begin. The writing drill sequence is listed in Table 7-2.

Another approach to writing treatment was developed by Haskins (1976). Her program employs a multimodality approach, emphasizing auditory and visual comprehension and retention, verbal cuing, and kin-

**Table 7-1.  Strengthening the Gestural Response**

1. Clinician gestures and says the word simultaneously.
2. Clinician says word, clinician and patient gesture simultaneously (clinician assistance with gesture may be required).
3. Patient imitates gesture.
4. Patient imitates gesture after enforced delay.
5. Patient gestures in response to auditory stimulus.
6. Patient gestures in response to auditory stimulus after enforced delay.
7. Patient gestures in response to written stimulus.
8. Patient gestures in response to written stimulus after enforced delay.
9. Patient writes word in response to gestural and auditory stimulus.
10. Patient gestures in response to appropriate question.

esthetic feedback. Haskins's program is presented here in a modified form, most notably by omitting oral spelling by the patient, writing words in a particular category, and having the patient generate and write a sentence using a word presented by the clinician. The steps in the program are listed in Table 7-3.

## Treating Drawing

When words or gestures fail them, people frequently resort to simple illustrations. Many globally aphasic patients retain some elementary ability to draw, and this ability can be enhanced in most of them.

Treatment for drawing begins by first having the patient copy simple geometric shapes. If these copies are not reasonable approximations, the patient is assisted in copying them until he or she can copy a reasonable approximation on his or her own. These simple shapes include a star, cone, rectangle, oval, and triangle. If the patient learns to draw these successfully, advance to more common objects, including house, tree, bottle, car, and ladder, employing the same procedure used in copying simple shapes.

Drawing is encouraged in later stages of treatment and is monitored frequently. It is an important part of a functional communication program called total communication. The use of drawing in this program is discussed in greater detail in a later section and in Chapter 8.

## Communication Boards

Communication boards seem to be the first thing nursing staff members and other hospital personnel think of when they discover that a patient

**Table 7–2.  Writing Drill for Aphasic Patients**

1. Tracing of single words with assistance if necessary. It is often a good idea to begin with large block letters stenciled or outlined letters.

2. Copying of single words.

3. Prolonged exposure (as long as the patient needs it) of the target word, with several repetitions of the auditory analogue.

4. Brief presentation of auditory and lexical stimulus, with written response.

5. Brief presentation of auditory and lexical stimulus, with imposed delay (5 to 15 seconds), then a written response.

6. Writing to dictation, with a return to previous levels at any point if necessary.

7. Writing to pictured presentation.

8. Writing in response to question (e.g. "What would you write if you were thirsty?" or "Write this person's name").

is unable to speak or gesture meaningfully. For some reason, the ability to point to pictures, to point to words, or to spell words with an alphabet board is thought to be an isolated skill unrelated to speaking, gesturing, or comprehension of language. Clinicians, of course, wish that were true. Many have found, however, that with appropriate training some globally aphasic patients can use a communication board effectively, provided that the message is simple and the listener is patient and insightful. Alphabet boards, or boards that contain only single words or ideas, generally are not effective for the globally aphasic patient. Some patients, however, make more effective use of boards containing both the picture and its written equivalent. Presentation of both pictures and words seems to enhance the saliency of the stimuli. Additional enhancement may be provided by constructing individualized communication boards, containing words or pictures that are particularly useful to that patient, and, if that fails or is not as rewarding as anticipated, the use of boards containing pictures of wife, children, familiar household objects, and personal objects. Pictures of items belonging to the patient can be taken with a camera that takes self-developing pictures and affixed to a board covered with acetate or acrylic.

Whichever type of board is chosen, training in its use is essential. Training should begin with a format similar to that used for natural language learning, in which initially only the target word is exposed. The clinician should repeat the stimulus, probably in sets of five, until the patient can point unfailingly to the named item. When that level is achieved, the item should be presented again, this time with approximately a 15 second delay.

The next step is to present one foil and again ask the patient to point to the target. This foil should be maximally differentiated from the

**Table 7–3.  Haskins's Writing Program for Aphasic Patients**

1. Clinician points to letters of the alphabet as the sound is produced and increases the number of letters in sequence as success is achieved.

2. Clinician points to printed words after synthesizing the sounds of the words into a whole (e.g., g-o, c-a-t), beginning with two sounds and gradually increasing the length of the words.

3. Patient points to the letter after the clinician names it, or the patient traces the letter after it is named.

4. Patient points to printed words after the clinician spells them, beginning with short, unrelated words that have varied spellings, and gradually increasing the complexity by selecting words with similar spellings.

5. Patient points to printed words after the clinician names them, beginning with four short, common words and increasing the display to ten more abstract words as the patient improves.

6. Patient copies letters of the alphabet, beginning with printed capital letters, then small (lower case) printed letters, eventually transcribing these to cursive letters if improvement permits.

7. Patient writes letters of the alphabet to dictation, beginning with the alphabet in serial order, then in random order.

8. Patient writes words to dictation. These words should be words that have been drilled in previous sequences (that is, by tracing, pointing, and so forth).

target, and it should not be an item presented anywhere else on the communication board.

When the patient can successfully point to the desired pictured object, the foil should be removed, and two items on the communication board are exposed. The clinician should present only the previously trained item first, in sets of five. When the patient is consistently successful, present the second item, again in sets of five. Do not alternate between items at this point. Gradually reduce the number of presentations, first to four, then to three, then to two. At this point, let the patient know clearly that the next item will be the foil. Again, as with the other item, gradually reduce the number of presentations. At this point, begin alternating between items, with two presentations for each. Allow the patient plenty of time to respond, and be certain that the item is presented clearly.

The same procedure should be followed for each of the items to be in the patient's core vocabulary. Performance often begins to falter, even after prolonged and intensive training, when five or more items are exposed, and there may be at least a temporary ceiling on the number of items that can be used on one board. One alternative is to use several boards, one containing pictures of family, another containing pictures of family and friends, and a third containing pictures of familiar household and personal objects.

This is a tedious process, but one that probably cannot be hurried. It may be best to limit this training to only part of each session.

## TREATING RECEPTIVE ABILITIES

### Total Physical Response

Asher (1981) published a provocative theory based in part on Piagetian views of how infants acquire language. Asher stated that adults find it easier to acquire a second language through similar conditions than by more traditional methods. He developed a program called Total Physical Response (TPR) to teach foreign languages. This program differs from more traditional approaches, according to Asher, because it takes a "right hemisphere first" approach and relies on physical response, first to demonstration by the instructor, and then to commands and instructions following the demonstration. In this method, the instructor speaks the foreign language to direct physical activities (e.g., "stand up," "sit down," or "Walk over to Amy and dance with her"). Asher found that novel commands are especially memorable if they are playful, bizarre, or even silly—for example, "Give me your wristwatch, walk around the table, and scream." We have not found any globally aphasic patients who could follow that command, but neither have we found any who could respond correctly to "Put the watch on the other side of the pencil and then turn over the card." Asher offered impressive data for his language program with adults. The notion is engaging and, at least in theory, potentially useful because of what clinicians know about the globally aphasic patient's ability to follow whole body (axial) commands, such as "push your chair back," "close the door," and even "Hand me my glasses over there on the desk."

An adequate data base has not yet been collected on experiments with this method, but preliminary results are promising, and the method is worthy of serious exploration.

More information is needed about whether this ability can be enlisted to improve comprehension in globally aphasic patients. It may be, however, that comprehension is more or less intact but the output modality cannot be harnessed.

### Playing Cards to Facilitate Comprehension

For some reason, playing cards, and patients' recognition and use of them, are among the most useful of stimuli. Patients often can recognize names that contain two salient features (for example, "queen of hearts"), differentiate cards by suit, and place cards in sequence when they are unable to perform similar tasks with other stimuli. A program has been formalized based on this peculiar ability. Many clinicians use some variation of this protocol and have found it useful. At its least effective, it seems to interest patients and hold their attention when other stimuli fail. Additionally, this program produces responses that seem to operate sequentially under proper stimulus control, and, although not all patients eventually achieve the highest levels of performance, portions of the program are useful at some stage for most patients.

The program begins with matching and sequencing of playing cards. At this level, matching is demonstrated by the clinician, who presents two cards that are maximally differentiated—for example, 2 of spades and ace of hearts. Stimulus control is important here, and the stimuli must be maximally differentiated by sound (name), by color, and by suit.

The clinician then demonstrates matching by placing an additional card (for example, the 4 of hearts) on the ace of hearts, then the 6 of spades on the 2 of spades. After several trials, the patient is asked to match cards as already demonstrated. Rather than introduce new cards at this stage it is advisable to use the same cards used in the demonstration. Several purposes seem to be accomplished by this task.

First, it seems to direct, orient, and alert the patient to treatment tasks by demanding some performance from him or her that he or she is capable of attaining. Second, it allows the clinician to make some determination about higher levels that might be possible. Third, it provides for small steps of increasing stimulus complexity that are easily controlled by the clinician. Finally, it seems to be effective, although its efficacy, or its usefulness to produce generalization to other tasks, has not been formally demonstrated with adequate controls.

In the third step, new cards are introduced, all of which are maximally differentiated. Criterion for success, and for advancement to more complex tasks, should be substantial, because the likelihood at this level for responding correctly by chance is high. Setting criterion at 90 percent correct reduces this likelihood.

When that criterion has been reached, usually for 20 or 30 trials, the fourth, fifth, and sixth steps can be introduced sequentially, maintaining the same stimulus controls. In these steps, increasing complexity is added first by increasing the number of foils, from two to three and finally to four, reducing the differentiation by color and then by suit. Additional complexity can be added by placing two like colors side-by-side rather than alternating them.

In the seventh step, the patient is asked to match cards by number, first in the same suit with one foil, next in the same suit with two and then three foils, and then in different suits with one, two, and finally three foils.

In the next step, the patient is asked to sequence cards, first with three numbers, then with four, and then with five. In the initial stage, sequencing should be within the same suit. In subsequent stages, suits should be varied, first maximally and then minimally.

In the second major level (a level that begins to tax comprehension rather than recognition), the patient is required first to listen to one unvarying command ("hand me") and then, as difficulty level increases, to differentiate by color, by number, and by suit, beginning with cards that are maximally differentiated and then using cards with decreasing differentiation. Begin this stage by presenting only one card, demonstrating the desired response. To ensure that the task is understood, present a minimum of five trials. Once the demonstration is complete, begin by presenting one foil, and asking the patient (for example), "Hand me the queen of hearts." At this level, it is probably not necessary to maintain such a rigid criterion for success and advancement to the next level. Seventy or 80 percent is probably adequate and probably ensures that the task has been learned well enough to advance to the next level.

In the next level, complexity is increased, alternating the commands. In the initial step, the patient is asked to "turn over" a card, identifying it from one foil. The task is first demonstrated by the clinician. Ten trials of each are presented. In the next step, the clinician alternates between "hand me the card" and "turn over the card," with five randomized trials of each in the one foil condition, five of each in the two foil condition, and five of each in the three foil condition.

In the next phase, only one foil is exposed, and the patient is asked (for example), "Put the queen of hearts on the ace of diamonds." Even though only one choice is possible, ten trials are recommended. Success at this level should advance the patient to the next two levels, with two, and then three, foils exposed.

In subsequent steps, complexity is increased by decreasing differentiation, by additional foils, by maximally alternating the commands, and by the addition of prepositions of place. The later phases are similar to the format for both the original *Token Test* (DeRenzi and Vignolo, 1962) and the *Revised Token Test* (McNeil and Prescott, 1978). In the final stage, three foils are exposed, and the commands maximally differentiate the cards. A summary of this format is shown in Table 7–4.

The procedure described here and in Table 7–4 may also be used as a supplemental evaluative measure. No normative data are available, and its concurrent validity has not been tested. The procedure may also be used as both a pretest (by excluding the one foil and demonstration

**Table 7–4.  Program Using Playing Cards for Aphasic Patients**

I.  Matching and Sequencing
   a.  Demonstration with alternating red and black suits, one foil.
   b.  Demonstration with alternating red and black suits, two foils.
   c.  Demonstration with alternating red and black suits, three foils.
   d.  Matching by suit with alternating red and black suits, two foils.
   e.  Matching by suit with alternating red and black suits, three foils.
   f.  Demonstration of matching by number with four cards, same suit and number.
   g.  Patient matching by number with four cards, same suit and number.
   h.  Demonstration of sequencing by suit, first with five cards of the same suit, then with five cards of four different suits.
   i.  Patient sequencing by suit, first with five cards of the same suit, then with five cards of four different suits.

II.  Comprehension and gestural response
   a.  Comprehension and gestural response of one command, with cards maximally differentiated by color, number, and suit. The command is "hand me."
   b.  Same as a, with two foils.
   c.  Same as a, with three foils.
   d.  Comprehension and gestural response of one command, with decreasing differentiation of cards.
   e.  Increasing complexity with redundant message
      (1)  Same as IIa, with one foil. Command here is "turn over." Then use two foils, and then three foils.
      (2)  Increasing complexity with redundant message. Two elements are involved here—for example, "Put the queen of hearts on the ace of spades."

III.  Comprehension with emphasis on adjectives and pronouns. Arrangement of the cards will vary with the stimulus.
   A.  1.  Pick up all of the cards.
       2.  Pick up all of the diamonds.
       3.  Pick up all of the 10s.
       4.  Pick up all of the diamonds.
       5.  Pick up all of the 2s.
       6.  Pick up all of the 4s.
       7.  Pick up the ace.
       8.  Pick up the 4.
       9.  Pick up the 6.
      10.  Pick up the 7.
   B.  Decreasing differentiation, two cards exposed, same number but different suit. The command is "hand me."
       1.  Same format, with two foils.
       2.  Same format, with three foils.
   C.  Decreasing differentiation, one foil, maximally differentiated; number, suit, and color of cards in random order. Varying comprehension and gestural requirements.
       1.  Turn over the ace of spaces.
       2.  Put the 4 of spades under the 7 of diamonds.
       3.  Put the ace of spaces on top of the 10 of diamonds.
       4.  Put the 3 of hearts above the 6 of clubs.
       5.  Put the 3 of clubs below the 6 of hearts.
       6.  Put the queen of diamonds to the left of the 9 of spades.
       7.  Put the ace of spaces to the right of the 9 of clubs.
       8.  Put the 2 of clubs beside the 9 of diamonds.
       9.  Put the ace of hearts over the 2 of spades.
      10.  Put the 5 of diamonds next to the jack of clubs.

conditions, as a treatment procedure, by changing the elements in the commands to similar elements) and as a posttest (by changing the commands again to those used in the pretest). All levels of course will not be appropriate for all patients. The hierarchy is unfortunately a concept, and not always a reality; a clinician's vision, despite optimism, should not extend beyond his or her goals.

The procedure is most efficiently implemented in a Base-10 format, with ten items to each Base-10.


## TRADITIONAL TREATMENT OF COMPREHENSION

Marshall (1979) notes that a number of factors must be controlled by the clinician to make the stimulus adequate and, of equal importance, to increase the probability that the response is adequate. These message delivery techniques have been reviewed and summarized elsewhere (most notably by Darley, 1976), but they are worth reviewing here because they increase the likelihood that not only the therapy used by clinicians, but their communication, with and for globally aphasic patients is successful.

**Rate of Speaking.** A slower rate of speaking has a beneficial effect on comprehension by aphasic patients.

**Pause Insertion.** Pause insertion involves the deliberate use of a brief pause, usually at a syntactical boundary. Pauses that separate messages into segments containing two or fewer bits of information are processed more efficiently by aphasic patients, but for some patients with auditory retention problems, requiring the patient to retain material for a longer period of time may have an adverse effect on comprehension.

**Alerting Signals.** Alerting signals prepare the patient for a forthcoming message and seem to improve the performance of severely aphasic patients. Different types of alerting signals do not differentially affect comprehension.

**Interstimulus Pause Time.** Interstimulus pause time refers to the insertion of time between stimulus presentations. Brief pauses between stimulus deliveries may prevent error or perseverative responses on subsequent stimulations.

**Response Time.** Response time refers to the extra time allowed to the patient to make a decision regarding a particular stimulus. Lengthening response time, and particularly allowing the patient to respond at his or her own rate, has been found to be beneficial to performance by aphasic patients on certain language tasks.

**Imposed Delay of Response.** Processing of a message may be facilitated by preventing the patient from responding immediately after delivery of the message. Some authorities have found that imposing delay may prevent subjects from making anticipatory errors.

**Stress.** In the broadest sense, stress refers to those suprasegmental features of speech that emphasize selected aspects of a verbal message. Perception of stress is a function of pitch, duration, and loudness, or a combination of these attributes. A number of authorities have found that perception of stress is relatively preserved in aphasia, and selective and appropriate use of stress may enhance comprehension. For example, comprehension may be facilitated by prolonging or accenting syllables, phonemes, or words to stress their importance.

**Stimulus Exposures.** Stimulus exposure refers to the number of stimuli to which the patient is exposed, including length of stimuli, competing stimuli, or additional stimuli from which the patient is to select one appropriate response.

**Semantic Field.** Semantic field refers to the semantic environment surrounding the stimulus. In general, the closer the stimuli are in meaning (for example, car, bus, truck, and taxi), the greater the difficulty the aphasic patient will have in identifying the target from those four choices. The more disparate the items (for example, car, soup, bed, and wrench), the greater the likelihood that the patient will make the correct choice.

Several other factors need to be considered in controlling the stimulus and, in effect, controlling response adequacy. These include the sometimes disastrous effects on performance of medications, illness, fatigue, depression, extraneous noise in the environment, and peripheral perceptual deficits.


## CLINICIAN CONTROLLED AUDITORY STIMULATION

Marshall (1979) has prepared a treatment package that takes into account many of the factors discussed earlier. His *Clinician Controlled Auditory Stimulation for Aphasic Adults* consists of a set of stimulus cards and a recording form. The cards are grouped and organized to allow the clinician to control the difficulty of the stimulus presented, which means, essentially, that it allows the clinician control over many of the factors discussed earlier. The recording form, for example, provides for specification of identifying information, message delivery techniques, and the documentation of responses to auditory stimulations.

The stimulus cards consist of 360 pictured nouns. They are divided into three 60-pair sets, permitting the exposure of two, four, or six pictures simultaneously. The cards are grouped to provide for control of the syllabic length, initial phoneme, and number of semantic and phonetically related stimuli presented. Using these stimuli, and combinations of them, stimuli can be presented that allow for minimal semantic relationship (e.g., broom and ring) or increased semantic relationship (e.g., hammer and nail, or banana and apple).

The recording form provides for identifying information and notation of psychological, situational, or physiological variables that may influence performance; space for task description, documenting use of message delivery techniques, recording of stimuli and responses to probes, and the coding of 80 stimuli and responses to the treatment task; and a summary of the patient's performance, assessment of results, and future planning.

Finally, Marshall's program (1979) allows for the recording of responses along an eight-step, multidimensional continuum, with 8 being an accurate, responsive, and prompt response, and 1 being a frank error, no response, or a rejection of the stimulus. This scoring system is shown in Table 7–5.

Use of these stimulus cards can permit the clinician to design tasks commensurate with the patient's needs and a variety of difficulty levels, including verbal and nonverbal responses—for example, identifying by name, by function, by combining identification of items by name and function; identification of items by preposition, or by description; auditory stimulation without visual cues; affirmative and negative questions; use of wh-questions; and complicated commands.

## Natural Language Learning

Natural language learning is a concept for learning languages that has its roots in "controlled auditory stimulation," which has been formalized by Winitz, Reeds, and Garcia (1975) for the teaching of foreign languages and first language learning. Generally, controlled auditory stimulation is taken to mean that verbal responses should be elicited but not forced. That is, individuals are provided with extensive practice in language comprehension, but speaking is neither trained nor required. The system developed by Winitz and colleagues makes two basic assumptions for natural language learning: that language is acquired through comprehension and that grammar becomes internalized through practice in problem solving.

Experience in language comprehension is believed by other authorities (Asher, 1981; Lenneberg, 1967) to be the primary avenue through which language is acquired, requiring that linguistic structures must be

**Table 7–5. Descriptive Category System for Use with Clinician Controlled Auditory Stimulation for Aphasic Adults**

| Score | Response |
|-------|----------|
| 8 | Accurate, responsive, prompt response |
| 7 | Accurate, responsive, minimally delayed response |
| 6 | Accurate, responsive, minimally delayed response |
| 5 | Accurate, responsive, self-corrected response |
| 4 | Accurate, responsive, but items are given out of sequence. For example, clinician says, "Point to the ball and the car" and the patient points to the car and the ball) |
| 3 | Accurate response after repetition of the stimulus |
| 2 | Related error (e.g., patient selects a semantically or phonetically related stimulus) |
| 1 | Frank error, no response, rejection of stimulus |

Note: The terms accurate, responsive, and prompt are used to refer to the rightness or correctness of a response, the ease with which the response is elicited, and the degree of immediateness (or latency). This usage is intended to parallel descriptions given earlier by Porch (1967).

understood before they can be stored in memory. Production of language is generally regarded as the outcome of experience in comprehension rather than a basic routine for establishing language.

Problem solving, as Winitz and associates (1975) use the term, refers to the conceptual operations necessary for language comprehension. Essentially, it refers to the solving of grammatical problems. In format, natural language learning paradigms are similar to many therapeutic endeavors. The individual is asked to listen to a word or phrase and then select from three or four pictures the one that accurately reflects the verbal stimulus, which may be more of a basic problem-solving strategy than a comprehension task. Because this task is relatively easy for aphasic patients and places limited demands on linguistic abilities, it is often a beginning for more complex tasks, which may involve increasing the choices, increasing the complexity of the stimulus, and so forth. This notion has an appealing logic to it. If we normally learn language through exposure and comprehension to stimuli, environmental and otherwise, perhaps aphasic patients should respond to similar learning paradigms. The one potential flaw to this notion, however, is that aphasic patients probably do not learn in the same ways because the mechanism they are attempting to learn with is not intact. It is known that aphasic patients do learn, and that their learning curve parallels that of normal people (Carson, Carson, and Tikofsky, 1968), but what is still not known is the internal strategies that must be employed, or the internal adjustments that must be made, to achieve these levels of learning. Until more has been determined, theoretical constructs with face validity must be tested empirically. The best of these stand up as useful therapies but may not stand up as useful explanations for models or explanations.

The theory of Winitz and colleagues (1975) was tested empirically by Kushner and Winitz (1977) with an aphasic patient. There are serious theoretical and methodological problems with the study, but it is nevertheless an important study because it proceeds from a logical, thoughtful theoretical construct, it was a well designed and appropriate probe measure applied systematically, and the authors realized its limitation.

Winitz and associates (1975) used this treatment approach with a 47 year old man with residual aphasia following a traumatic injury and subsequent left temporal lobectomy. He was initially tested at 1 month post onset with several speech and language measures; his overall performance on the PICA placed him at the 24th percentile for aphasic adults. Treatment apparently began almost immediately.

In this treatment program, 19 different common nouns are represented graphically and are repeated frequently in 106 frames. Items of increasing difficulty are systematically introduced. The first frame, for example, consists of only one item, "pencil." The patient is instructed to point to the correct picture after the clinician produces a single isolated noun. Correct responses led to presentation of the next frame, which again contained only the single picture. When the patient produced an incorrect response, the stimulus item was repeated again, and the clinician pointed to the picture.

After several frames of correct responses, a second word (for example, "shirt") is added, and successive pictures are added until all frames are filled.

The patient was required to point to the correct response and was not asked to imitate. No attempt was made to control his verbalizations when they occurred. Each session was 30 minutes long, which was generally sufficient time to complete all 106 frames. Treatment sessions were held several times each week, and the patient received no other treatment during this time.

In all, the patient received 21 treatments in what appears to be a natural withdrawal design. The results are striking not so much because of his improvement on the comprehension tasks (approximately 78 percent to 100 percent over the duration of the study), but because of his improvement on production of the treated nouns, which improved from 20 percent correct to 100 percent correct during the same time. Performance also improved on all generalization measures (e.g., PICA and *Token Test)* and this improvement continued during the no-treatment periods, providing some evidence for the occurrence of generalization.

Kushner and Winitz (1975) believe that their results speak for generalization and to the effects of treatment and not to spontaneous recovery because performance declined somewhat during the period of no treatment. They conclude that controlled auditory stimulation can be "reinterpreted to mean the systematic teaching of language comprehension. Success in production should reflect achievement in comprehension" (p. 304).

It may also be that the stimuli, which are line drawings of objects contained in a display with narrow perimeters, enhances visual recognition. Helm-Estabrooks (1981) notes that pointing to objects in the environment may require better visual search, selection, attention, and verbal memory skills than does pointing to a more limited array of pictured items, and that there is some evidence to suggest that patients are better able to point to pictures presented one on a card than to pictures grouped together on a single card. Her study of 21 patients with severe auditory comprehension deficits suggests that some patients have difficulty *finding* objects rather then recognizing them, and also that therapy might be directed toward improving visual search skills, beginning with the condition that elicited the best performance and gradually moving toward the most difficult condition. It is possible, based on this evidence, that the structure of natural language learning facilitates *both* auditory comprehension and visual search skills.

## TREATING SPEECH

Despite the most relentless and vigorous therapeutic assault, speech will not become an independent, functional mode of communication for the globally aphasic patient, but even several useful words, used in conjunction with other forms of communication or, rarely, used independently, may make a tremendous difference in a patient's functional abilities. In general, however, speech drill should be reserved for those patients who show the most potential for it. Clinicians should not equate recurring utterances with involuntary utterances. Recurring utterances are rarely useful unless the intonation that accompanies them is variable, appropriate, and predictable. In the author's clinic, speech drill is generally reserved for those patients who can repeat single words (and some can repeat an occasional phrase) however sporadically. We do not anticipate generalization to other stimuli, situations, or settings, and are not disappointed when this does not occur in our testing. Neither, however, do we reject it when it appears. Generally, our stimuli are as salient and as differentiated as we can make them. Specific examples of stimuli, and patients' response to them as stimuli, accompany the case presentations in Chapter 8. In general, however, we follow a protocol that capitalizes and builds on the ability to repeat, moving through successive stages of imitation, imitation with delay, reading, and use in appropriate situations. Because we are reluctant to work solely on speech, and because our ultimate goal is functional, or total, communication, we incorporate other modalities into the drill. Treatment becomes, in essence, multimodality treatment with an emphasis, depending on strengths and weaknesses, on one modality or another. Our modified eight step task continuum is outlined in Table 7–6.

## VOLUNTARY CONTROL OF INVOLUNTARY UTTERANCES (VCIU)

In 1980, Helm and Barresi presented a seemingly novel approach to aphasia therapy. What they actually did was systematize and formalize an approach to treatment presented in print by at least one author (Goda, 1962) and probably used in a less systematic manner by countless clinicians who were beguiled by spontaneous utterances that frequently were not appropriate for the situation in which they were uttered but were potentially appropriate in other situations.

What captured the imagination of clinicians was that if those utterances could be brought under voluntary control, or if patients could be taught to remember those utterances and use them in appropriate instead of inappropriate situations, communication would be enhanced significantly. Superficially, that notion has a great deal of merit. What can be produced spontaneously can at least potentially be produced volitionally. Unfortunately, at least for most of us, those utterances have remained elusive, perhaps because remaining neural mechanisms do not allow for the control and inhibition required to produce them volitionally under traditional treatment regimens, or because other neural mechanisms are not responsive.

Helm and Barresi (1980) applied their program to the verbal output of three very different aphasic patients. These patients were not classifiable by any traditional aphasia nosology and could probably not be classified as having global aphasia. All three patients, however, were severely impaired in verbal output, all three had moderately intact auditory comprehension, and none of the patients had responded to the "most robust" treatment efforts. Lesion location and profiles of deficits differed for these patients. One patient was a left-handed man who suffered a right hemisphere lesion that left him severely aphasic and with left hemiplegia.

**Table 7–6.  Speech Drill Hierarchy—Modified**

| | |
|---|---|
| Step 1. | Clinician produces the target. |
| Step 2. | Clinician produces the target three times, pausing between each. |
| Step 3. | Clinician and patient produce target utterance simultaneously. |
| Step 4. | Patient repeats target utterance after clinician's utterance while clinician mimes utterance. |
| Step 5. | Clinician produces target utterance and patient repeats. No other cues. |
| Step 6. | Clinician produces target utterance and patient repeats it several times with no intervening cues. |
| Step 7. | Patient reads target utterance presented on card. |
| Step 8. | Patient copies target utterance. |
| Step 9. | Patient produces target utterance after 5 second exposure to target. |
| Step 10. | Patient is presented with card, card is withheld, and patient is asked to produce target utterance. |
| Step 11. | Patient responds with target utterance when asked an appropriate question by clinician. |

This program begins by presenting the patient with printed words or phrases which he or she has been heard to utter during the formal evaluation, or with emotionally laden words which appear to be easier for aphasic patients to read aloud than concrete and nonemotional words. If the patient is immediately able to read the word or phrase correctly, it is printed on an index card to be used for self-monitored drills. If, instead of reading the word as printed, the patient utters a different *real* word, the original word is discarded and the patient's newest word is substituted. In this stage of the program, the patient cannot make an error unless he or she produces a neologism or produces no response at all. If the patient struggles with the target word, treatment is not focused on this word. Oral reading of the word lists then gives way to more volitional, propositional use of the target words through more traditional, response naming and confrontation naming tasks, then expository speech tasks, and finally conversation. These steps are not outlined, but presumably an eight-step task continuum, such as the one proposed by Rosenbek et al. (1973) or a response-contingent small step (RCSST) program, such as the one proposed by Bollinger and Stout (1974), would be appropriate.

Their patients made significant gains on four naming subtests of the BDAE: responsive naming, confrontation naming, body part naming, and animal naming. The first patient eventually generated a lexicon of 290 words and phrases, which were read correctly and could be used in natural speech settings, but his oral reading scores on the BDAE remained unchanged.

The second patient, who had virtually no naming skills prior to VCIU treatment, improved on each subtest, with the greatest gains occurring on confrontation naming. Although his pre- and posttreatment reading scores remained unchanged, he was eventually able to read 271 words aloud and to read phrases with "good consistency" and use these in a conversational setting.

The third patient improved in all but body part naming, although his BDAE oral reading scores never exceeded the three words he read aloud before treatment. Nevertheless, his lexicon grew to 259 words and phrases that he was eventually able to use voluntarily for daily communicative purposes.

Helm and Barresi (1980) do not tell us what constitutes a "conversational" situation. Presumably, the situations were contrived by the clinician or the clinician covertly transcribed the patient's speech in conversational settings. Many of the words the patients produced do appear to be useful in conversational contexts. Interestingly, the words appear to have little in common, and few of them are "emotionally laden." The exceptions appear to be "dammit," "good," "hello," "hi," possibly "I don't know," "love," "money," "mad," "no," "okay," "shame," "shit," "thanks," "that's right," "what," and "yes." Most are common nouns, with no proper nouns (with one possible exception, "Coke"). Of the 122 words in their master list, 22 may be used as verbs; the remainder are common nouns, adverbs, adjectives, pronouns, and declaratives. Of the 122 words, 28 were common to all three patients (examples are "Coke," "I don't know," "love," "money," and "OK").

All patients eventually moved to another form of treatment, one in a syntax program in which the phrases and sentences were composed of words from the patient's VCIU list, and another in a form of Melodic Intonation Therapy (MIT) which draws on the patient's VCIU core vocabulary.

Globally aphasic patients produce few real, spontaneous utterances. They may produce an occasional expletive, occasionally their spouse's name, or the name of a few common objects or places. There does not seem to be any commonality to these productions, but most of them could probably be predicted. When they are used, they are often at least tangentially appropriate. A patient who remembers that he has to take his medication, has to go to the toilet, or needs a ride home may say "Mary!" in an attempt to convey any one or more of those situations. "Mary" is of course tangentially related because Mary is the one who administers his medication, or makes certain he gets to the bathroom, and takes him home from therapy. Knowing which of those is the intended communication requires skill, perseverance, and a lot of questions requiring "yes" and "no" answers. Appropriate, volitional production of two or three appropriate words, "Mary," "pills," and "ride," would make the communication process immensely simpler. If the patient's performance suggests that perhaps he or she is just a bit better in speech, or if it demonstrates the potential for learning a few words, VCIU is a potentially useful technique.

## TOTAL COMMUNICATION

Total communication is a term that has its genesis in pragmatic approaches to treatment. "Doing what works," or enhancing the abilities already possessed by the patient, is an approach most clinicians resort to eventually and is the heart of total communication programs. The total communication approach recognizes residual skills and capitalizes on them, encouraging the use of any or all channels of communication. Drawing, writing, pointing, gesturing, communication boards, and such devices as memory joggers—with familiar names, data, and locations included in it—are effective communication devices. Their use should not only be encouraged, but trained.

Earlier discussion of specific treatment techniques were based on the assumption that no single communicative modality or device will meet the communication needs of every globally aphasic patient. The goal of each of these techniques should be their incorporation into a program of total communication. How the clinician incorporates these newly learned, refocused, and residual skills will depend upon the patient's unique abilities, preferences, and needs. In general, however, once the patient has achieved some basic skill in one or two modalities, at least part of every treatment session should be devoted to a program designed to facilitate, stimulate, and encourage communication through those channels, in a format similar to that used for PACE. Following each communicative interaction—for example, around a theme prompted by a patient's interest, hobby, or background—specific drill on key words or devices used in the communication can be drilled employing one of the sequences already discussed.

In Chapter 8, specific and individualized programs are described for three very different globally aphasic patients. In a very general sense, however, the programs followed the following sequence:

1. Evaluation of residual skills and deficits.
2. Training to stabilize equivocal "yes" and "no" responses.
3. Writing drill.
4. Pointing drill.
5. Gestural drill.
6. Drill in use of objects as descriptors.
7. Speech drill.
8. Auditory comprehension drill.

# Chapter **8**

# Case Illustrations

The three case illustrations that follow represent three very different patients. The evolution of their aphasias, treatment requirements, backgrounds, motivation, and performance profiles differed. The single common factor that unites them is their global aphasia. That they have overcome, to some extent, their tremendous deficits and persevere in the face of an occasionally hostile and frequently bewildering world is a tribute to their spirit and resilience. This chapter is dedicated to these patients, and to their supporters—if their faith ever wavered, they never let it show.

In the early stages of recovery from a severe central nervous system trauma, patients frequently appear to be confused and are the victims of both their transient confusion and the permanent effects of their injury. It is conceivable that at some level they realize this. They fight our efforts to treat them, perhaps partly because through the curtains of their confusion they realize the severity of their deficits and their inability to control events. They appear to resent our intrusion, possibly because they believe that, with time, the curtain will lift and things will once again be the same. Eventually the curtain *will* lift but the scene and the soundtrack will never again be the same. In milder forms of aphasia, these initial deficits are profoundly frightening (Moss, 1972). We can only surmise that the enormity of the situation to the globally aphasic person is devastating.

Families are equally traumatized. Only the patient's appearance, voice, and an occasional idiosyncratic gesture hauntingly reveal the person they knew. Eventually, many of the traits that made the patient unique do return. We, however, know they will not all return. We know that a patient's personality will be altered; he or she will probably be less agreeable and more impatient. These deficits will irrevocably change the nature of all previous close relationships. We know this, but part of our obligation to the patient is not to reveal it, at least at this juncture.

Speech pathologists generally are not trained psychotherapists, yet we know a few of the guidelines: Be realistic, be firm, do not hedge, and do not allow your optimism or your pity to color your interpretation of events or your prognosis. We understand disordered behavior better than we understand normal behavior. We understand probabilities because of what we have read, what we have learned from our teachers, and what we have learned from our patients. If we are insightful and attentive, we have also learned that counseling the family of a severely aphasic patient requires a special skill. This skill is not one that has been taught us, and perhaps it cannot be taught. What we do mostly is react to the situation and serve as a sounding board. There are few hard and fast rules. Those that seem to be generally immutable, however, are the following:

1.  Remember that the family and the patient are grieving, and that grief colors the reactions and attitudes of even the most stable and realistic people.
2.  Remember that although we are the speech and language experts, the family are the experts with regard to the particular patient. They have known him or her and have lived with him or her much longer than we have known the patient.
3.  Remember that the family will doubt us, at least initially, because they need to. They need, at this point, to believe that everything will be all right, and that the healing effects of time will return everything to the status of yesterday.
4.  Remember that stroke to most people is an arcane and terrifying mystery. But people recover from other illnesses, and so they believe stroke should be no exception.
5.  Remember that our trained objectivity is an advantage that the family does not have, and should not have, at this point. The early stages of recovery should be filled with optimism, encouragement, and stimulation if the patient will allow it.
6.  Remember that, unless the information to be communicated is crucially important, there is little harm in allowing the family to believe that the patient *does* understand much of what is said to him, and that his shrugs, gestures, and verbal responses are meaningful and appropriate.
7.  Remember that families are as intelligent as we are, and that on crucial issues, the family is likely to take as much care as we will.

8.  Remember that, if we do our job properly, if we are wise, and if we are available, we can lead the family to a fuller understanding of the disorder in general and of its manifestations in that patient.

Case histories tend to be showcases for treatments that worked and patients who got better. Unfortunately, many patients do not get better despite the clinician's best efforts. It is important to know about these patients as well as the patients who do get better, because they are reminders that both clinicians and treatments are fallible. They also remind aphasiologists of how primitive treatments frequently are, and of how much still needs to be done.

## CHRONIC GLOBAL APHASIA

Mr. Loman is a 76 year old man who was in robust physical health until January of 1984, when he suffered a left hemisphere CVA. Neurologic and brain imaging tests revealed an extensive left hemisphere lesion involving the distribution of the left middle cerebral artery. In addition he was severely hemiplegic, with decreased sensation and a right visual field deficit (homonymous hemianopsia).

Formal speech and language testing was begun four days post onset. The results of the evaluation, which found Mr. Loman to be globally aphasic, follow:

**Listening.** Listening was severely involved. There is no evidence of the ability to understand even simple commands or yes-no questions.

**Reading.** Reading was severely involved. Mr. Loman appeared to recognize his name when given two choices, but his performance on a pointing task was highly variable. When given a group of three choices, he correctly pointed to the month and year on one occasion but could not do so later.

**Writing.** Writing was severely involved even for copying. The patient could copy portions of his name following some practice, but writing was perseverative, consisting primarily of E's and S's or unintelligible strokes.

**Speaking.** Speaking was severely involved. There was no evidence of ability to speak spontaneously or to repeat the days of the week, numbers, or other automatic phrases. The only vocalization heard was an approximation of the number "one."

**Object Recognition and Function.** Mr. Loman did not demonstrate consistent recognition of familiar objects such as "knife" or "comb," and he could not use objects functionally.

**Impressions.** Severe, global aphasic impairment across all modalities, with no evidence of peaks in performance.

## Plan

1. See the patient daily to provide speech and language stimulation.
2. Try to improve communication abilities using speech and gestural tasks.
3. Try use of a communication board, although it is suspected at this point that it will not help.
4. Suggestions for communicating with a severely aphasic patient will be posted on the patient's door, and a briefer list will be attached to his wheelchair.

**Suggestions.** Given the severity of this patient's deficits it would be both prudent and kind not to push communication. If he is to evolve, we will see the beginnings of that evolution in the next few weeks: he will respond more appropriately and with more spontaneity, will be more alert and responsive to his surroundings and to familiar environment, faces, objects, and voices, and will show us when our attempts to communicate make more sense to him.

No formal testing was done in the early stages of his recovery. The immediate objectives were to improve his ability to respond with "yes" or "no," assess his potential for learning to communicate with a modified communication board, and facilitate and stimulate auditory comprehension.

Treatment began by baselining the patient's responses to four tasks: pointing to the appropriate picture on his communication board (12 items) to lexical stimuli alone; to auditory stimuli alone; and to combined auditory and lexical stimuli; answering "yes" or "no" to a series of biographical questions. The baseline was 3 percent for auditory stimuli alone, 13 percent for lexical alone, 40 percent for combined auditory and lexical stimuli and 30 percent for "yes" and "no."

Treatment for each of those four tasks took most of the session. Some writing was also incorporated into the "point to _____ " treatment. Answering "yes" and "no" was the first priority. Because the patient's gestures were equivocal and his verbal responses unintelligible, we tried to inhibit those verbalizations initially.

The program began by asking him, for example, "Is your name Emil?" The patient's response generally was incorrect initially. When it was, the clinician would ask him to stop, model the appropriate gesture for him, physically assist him with the gesture several times accompanied by our model, pause, ask the question again, and repeat the process if necessary. Our reinforcement was immediate.

These responses were the focus of treatment during both sessions each day. We usually tested daily and alternated the time of day for our probes. The Base-10 shown in Figure 8-1 is a testimony to both our tenacity and the resistance of his aphasia to our ministrations. We were encouraged initially because Mr. Loman improved steadily over the first two sessions, slipped a bit, and climbed steadily to a high of 70 percent correct. We would have been pleased with that level. Unfortunately, for reasons we never understood and which were apparently unrelated to his physical condition, that improvement was ephemeral, and performance declined steadily despite continued treatment.

Four additional probes are not shown on the graph. Two occurred immediately following the last probe shown. Performance on those two again ascended to 30 percent. Six months later, Mr. Loman again achieved a high of 70 percent, but did not hold these gains, and one month later he returned to near baseline levels.

Our program to improve his ability to use the communication board began with tracing; copying with assistance; copying without assistance; clinician pointing to object and saying the appropriate word; patient

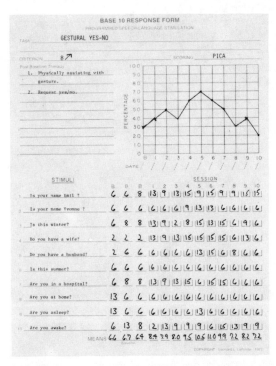

**Figure 8–1.** Base-10 response form for gestural "yes" and "no."

pointing to the object; and copying again. The communication board contained both the picture and, below it, the lexical stimulus. Our probes for the three conditions were administered less frequently, but with similar effect. As shown in Figures 8-2 and 8-3, improvements were unspectacular.

We persisted in attempts to treat these communication skills because Mr. Loman had demonstrated an inability to communicate in any other modality and even lacked the promise of being able to do so, and we believed it was his only hope for even fragmentary communication. We justified our persistence because it was our only link. When both we and our patient tired of the tediousness of the drill and the lack of progress on all but more simple and fun tasks, such as playing "21," matching cards by suit, working on a computer matching program, and attempting to use a simplified communication board functionally, we unanimously agreed to end his ordeal and let him get on with his life.

Mr. Loman returned for reevaluation several months later. His initial PICA score had improved from the 3rd percentile to the 6th, but with no significant improvement being seen in any modality. He enjoyed

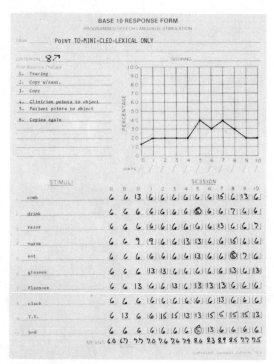

**Figure 8-2.** Base-10 response form—pointing responses to lexical stimuli on communication board.

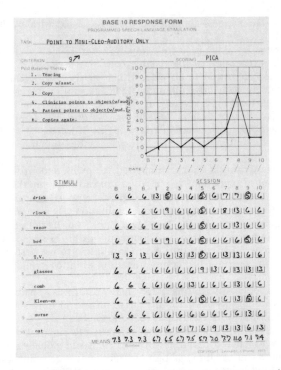

**Figure 8–3.** Base-10 response form—pointing responses to auditory stimuli on communication board.

a robust good health, although his severe hemiplegia confined him to a wheelchair. His wife reported no major difficulties in communicating with him, probably because his needs are simple and those he cannot provide for himself are anticipated. He attends to many of his needs independently. The results of our last evaluation show failure to improve on traditional tests, as does our summary of that evaluation (Figs. 8–2 and 8–3):

Mr. Loman is a 76 year old man who suffered a left hemisphere CVA on January 15, 1984. At that time he was diagnosed as globally aphasic without performance peaks in any modality. Since that time, his wife reports few changes in his communication abilities. However, she did report that he has been taken off all medications. The results of our reevaluation are outlined in the following paragraphs.

*Listening:* Listening is severely impaired. There is little evidence that Mr. Loman understands simple commands, and his understanding of yes-no questions is poor. He is unable to point to pictures of named objects predictably. He interacts appropriately and is blessed with excellent pragmatic skills.

*Speaking:* Speaking is severely impaired. Mr. Loman's only spontaneous speech is repetition of the syllable /ou/. He uses this in a variety of situations and, according to his wife, with a variety of different intonation patterns, which frequently communicate his general intent.

*Reading:* Reading is severely impaired. On the first three subtests of the *Reading Comprehension Battery for Aphasia* Mr. Loman scored a total of 18 of 30 correct compared with his score of 19 of 30 correct approximately 1 month post onset. He was unable to complete any additional items.

*Writing:* Writing is severely impaired. Copying and writing to dictation consisted of repetitions of "E" and unidentifiable marks.

*Other:* Overall, Mr. Loman now is more responsive, interacting more readily with the clinician than at earlier evaluation. He also produces more distinct gestural responses for "yes" and "no," but he does not use these accurately and uses the head nod commonly as his response in all situations. He made no attempt during this evaluation to use gestures to communicate. In general, his communication abilities remain extremely limited.

He was cooperative during our evaluation but was apparently anxious to leave, wheeling his chair toward the door several times. His apparent lack of interest in working with us remains unchanged.

*Impressions:* Mr. Loman has changed very little since our initial evaluation at approximately 1 month post onset. He is still globally aphasic, with severe involvement of all modalities. He does appear generally a little more responsive, and he demonstrates quicker, more differentiated, and accurate "yes" and "no" responses to simple questions. Some globally aphasic patients begin to show improvements in language comprehension and use at 6 months post onset or later, but our retesting shows no signs of this for Mr. Loman. His prognosis for significant improvement is poor, but continued small gains in functional communication, especially in very specific situations, can be expected. Owing to his lack of improvement and his apparent lack of interest in working on his speech and language, long-term speech treatment is not recommended. If it is consistent with his overall plan of medical management, we will follow him during this hospitalization, counsel his wife about his communicative abilities, and provide general language stimulation and facilitation.

## SEVERE, GLOBAL APHASIA WITH GRADUAL, MODEST IMPROVEMENT

Mr. Cross is a 62 year old man who suffered a left hemisphere CVA on November 3, 1980, which left him with a severe right flaccid hemiparesis, a right central facial weakness, and a right homonymous hemianopsia. His history was significant for myocardial infarction, angina pectoris, atrial fibrillation, and alcohol abuse. A brain scan administered on December 4, 1980, demonstrated decreased perfusion in the territory of the left middle cerebral artery. The static images also demonstrated an irregular region of increased tracer uptake confined to the territory of the left middle cerebral artery. The radiologist's impression was of extensive left temporoparietal infarct. A CT scan, administered the same day, revealed an area of abnormality in the distribution of the anterior and deep branches of the left middle cerebral artery. More fine-tuned analyses, which might have revealed the volume of this lesion, were not done. This scan was consistent with the brain scan and was suggestive of a subacute infarct. An electroencephalogram administered several days later showed slowing of the entire left cerebral hemisphere. The neurologist's impression: a massive lesion of the left temporal and parietal lobes, extending into the frontal lobe, in all likelihood caused by a thrombolic episode involving the distribution of the left middle cerebral artery.

Mr. Cross was referred for occupational, physical, and speech treatment, and our testing began 2 weeks post onset. At that time formal testing was impossible. Mr. Cross was irritable and combative and resisted our attempts to assess his deficits formally. Our consultation summary revealed the inadequacies, because it was brief, and it probably reflected more of what we knew about severe aphasia and the odds again significant recovery from such a massive lesion than it said about Mr. Cross:

62 year old man who suffered an apparent left CVA on November 3, 1980 which left him speechless and hemiplegic. Our testing reveals the following:

*Understanding:* Patient can inconsistently follow a few commands, such as "close your eyes," but follows no pointing commands. Yes-no responses are inconsistent, and he is probably operating at about a chance level in answering yes-no questions.

*Reading:* Patient rejects all reading tasks.

*Writing:* There is no evidence that he can copy or write even his name spontaneously.

*Speaking:* Patient did not speak except to say "yeah" at our first evaluation. We could elicit no automatic speech nor any serial speech, such as counting. He is essentially speechless.

*Impressions:* Global aphasia. The patient's prognosis is poor unless he begins to evolve in the next 2 weeks. We have begun twice daily treatments, including general stimulation and facilitation, a trial with a language board, and gestural training as an alternative mode of communication. He will benefit from

1.  As much stimulation as possible so long as people talk slowly with normal loudness, and one at a time.
2.  A combination of speech and demonstration.

3. Being treated as normally as possible—for example, being asked yes-no questions to answer.
4. Encourage his own gesturing in real-life situations.

Our expectations are that comprehension will continue to improve. Ward staff personnel can check his comprehension, particularly for more important communications about activities and needs of daily living, by asking first the desired question and then a question with opposite answer—for example, "Is your name Walt?" and then "Is your name Felicity?" If the patient answers "yes" to both questions, he could be playing the averages. We also expect that he will learn to copy and learn to read some single words.

We appreciate the staff's and family's concern about, and frustration with, the patient's severely diminished ability to communicate. We share these frustrations and concerns. Unfortunately, there is no easy and sure way to elicit functional communication. The patient is unable to write and may never be a functional writer again. Because his language is impaired, he will have as much difficulty spelling, pointing to the words he wants, or gesturing in a meaningful way as he does in writing. For these reasons, a functional communication board or a set of usable gestures are impossible for the foreseeable future. We hope this will not always be the case. For the time being, staff members, patient, and family will ensure the least traumatic communication by following the guidelines for communicating with a severely aphasic patient attached to his door and by being patient, optimistic, and realistic. In addition to our continued evaluation and treatment procedures to achieve some functional means of communication, we will begin counseling his family.

Mr. Cross's family was bright, patient, optimistic, and numerous. They visited the patient frequently, they accompanied him to his therapies, and they spoke privately to his therapists. We counseled them, encouraged them to stimulate and facilitate the patient's responses, showed them how, taught them about aphasia and their father's illness, and began to reveal some of his very poor prognosis. This prognosis became clearer as formal testing progressed.

We began formal testing at approximately 1 month post onset, not because there is anything magic about this particular time, but because that was when he was ready and because clinicians seem able to remember 1 month increments more easily than other increments.

We administered the *Porch Index of Communicative Ability* (PICA). Based on even our limited exposure to Mr. Cross, we were not surprised by our results. Average performance on the 18 subtests was 5.83, a score that placed him at the 8th percentile for aphasic adults. The mean of his nine highest subtests was 7.80 and the mean of his nine lowest subtests was 3.85. Based on these figures alone, performance at 6 months post onset could be projected to be at the 19th percentile. Even the most optimistic projection was for a global aphasia that would evolve slowly and incompletely. A summary of Mr. Cross's modality and variability scores (Table 8-1) and an individualized Ranked Response Summary (Fig. 8-4).

Table 8–1.  PICA Scores at One Month Post Onset

| Modality | Mean Score | Percentile | Mean Variability |
|----------|-----------|-----------|------------------|
| Overall | 5.83 | 8 | 18.3 |
| Writing | 4.55 | 12 | 2.0 |
| Copying | 6.00 | 8 | 40.0 |
| Reading | 6.15 | 13 | 23.5 |
| Pantomime | 4.45 | 5 | 15.5 |
| Verbal | 3.43 | 8 | 8.3 |
| Auditory | 6.70 | 8 | 48.0 |
| Visual | 13.25 | 8 | 17.5 |
| Highs | 7.80 | 8 | |
| Lows | 3.85 | 8 | |

Total Variability: 330
Mean Variability: 16.67
Six Month Prediction: 19th percentile

Analysis of subtest and item scores suggest that Mr. Cross's poorest performance occurred on gestural, verbal, and writing tasks. A ranked response summary of performance by easiest to most difficult tasks appears in Figure 8–4. The patient's best performance occurred on tests requiring reading, auditory comprehension, matching, imitation, and copying. Misleading subtest scores are those in which he rejected all items. Mr. Corss's mean score on subtest D, for example, is 5.0 because he rejected all items. On subtest E, however, mean performance was 4.4, but, although his responses were generally unintelligible, he attempted all tasks, and two of his responses were intelligible but wrong. Samples of Mr. Cross's writing appear in Figure 8–5.

The results of this test provided us with several useful pieces of information. First, the results showed that despite the severity of his aphasia, the patient was willing to tolerate almost 60 minutes of what for him were very difficult tasks, requiring attention, concentration, and resource allocation. Second, they gave us a solid baseline with which to compare future performance and a measure of generalization. Third, they told us, at least in a very general sense, what he could do and what he could not do at all, and that he did not benefit from repetitions or more direct cues. Fourth, the results provided us with a prognosis for future performance. The prospect of spending the rest of one's days at the 19th percentile is not an enviable one, but the variability of this patient's performance, which was unusual in global aphasia, also suggested that if all of the therapists did their jobs, he should do better than that. We also suspected that the 6 month prediction was conservative, because Mr. Cross might do better the second 6 months. Finally, the results provided us with direction for more fine-tuned testing and some direction for treatment.

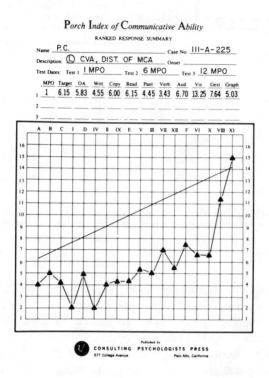

**Figure 8–4.** Graphic summary of performance on the 18 subtests of the PICA.

We administered three more tests. Because spontaneous speech was all but impossible for this patient, we did not do any further speech testing, but we did assess oral, nonverbal movements. Allowing for his difficulty in comprehension and a mild and improving right facial weakness but relatively well preserved abilities to imitate and repeat, we found he had a significant oral, nonverbal apraxia. He performed only one of ten tasks correctly: he was able to open his mouth. He was unable to protrude his tongue, bare his teeth, or purse his lips. Limb praxis was strikingly impaired. He performed only three of the ten tasks correctly, and those were to imitation.

We administered the *Reading Comprehension Battery for Aphasia* because we have found that it has a hierarchy of difficulty, that it is relatively quick, and that it provides useful information to be incorporated into treatment. Performance was surprisingly good on the first three subtests, which require matching of one of three foils to a picture of the object. Mr. Cross's scores were 7, 8, and 6. Performance dropped off substantially after that, however. On subtest 4, a test of functional sentence reading, only one response was correct. He identified five of ten synonyms correctly, but none of his responses to any of the items on the remaining five subtests—requiring functional reading of sentence and paragraph material—were correct.

We administered Raven's *Coloured Progressive Matrices* (Raven, 1962) because we have found it to be sensitive to the deficits in global aphasia, to be useful as one of a set of predictors, and to be a sensitive measure of physiological improvement over time. Mr. Cross scored 12 correct of 36 possible, which placed him below the 10th percentile for both normal men his age and patients with left hemisphere lesions and aphasia. We did no further formal testing at that time. We believed we had a fairly complete and accurate picture of his abilities as well as his deficits, and we were ready to formulate some treatment goals.

Because Mr. Cross's auditory comprehension was relatively well preserved (mean scores of 6.7 on both auditory subtests), we believed that he could begin to establish the foundation for some basic communication by listening to questions and responding with "yes" and "no." This procedure is limited because our imaginations are limited, because we miss a crucial event in the process, or because the patient desires something out of context or unrelated to current events; yet it provides very close to a normal communicative exchange. We had found, however, that "yes" and "no" responses were inconsistent and equivocal, and Mr. Cross frequently nodded for "yes" but said "no," or shook his head for negation and said "yes." We knew that his auditory comprehension was severely compromised, yet on formal tests of auditory comprehension we found reason for optimism.

On subtest VI, the more difficult of the two primary auditory tests, two of Mr. Cross's responses were correct. He required a repetition of one question and self-corrected another. We were impressed with the self-correction because it suggested a comprehension and self-monitoring uncommon in global aphasia. Mr. Cross produced one correct response, although delayed, on the less difficult subtest. The range of his correct responses, then, told us that his responses were not always hasty and ill-considered, that he had the capacity for self-correction, and that he benefited from controlled repetition. We predicted that, with appropriate treatment and under the proper conditions, the majority of his responses to simple auditory stimuli would be correct, allowing for an occasional repetition of instructions. Our first goal was stabilizing the yes-no response to auditory stimulation. A secondary goal, and one that could be addressed simultaneously, was to improve auditory comprehension.

Our ultimate goal was to make Mr. Cross a functional communicator within the limitations imposed on him by his physiological recovery.

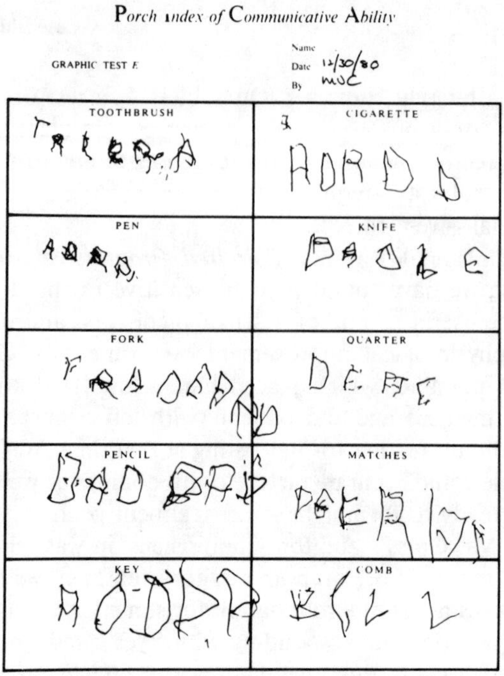

Porch Index of Communicative Ability

GRAPHIC TEST E

Name
Date 12/30/80
By MJC

| TOOTHBRUSH | CIGARETTE |
|---|---|
| *(handwritten)* | *(handwritten)* |
| PEN | KNIFE |
| *(handwritten)* | *(handwritten)* |
| FORK | QUARTER |
| *(handwritten)* | *(handwritten)* |
| PENCIL | MATCHES |
| *(handwritten)* | *(handwritten)* |
| KEY | COMB |
| *(handwritten)* | *(handwritten)* |

Porch Index of Communicative Ability

GRAPHIC TEST D

Name
Date 1/30/80
By MJC

Figure continued on following page

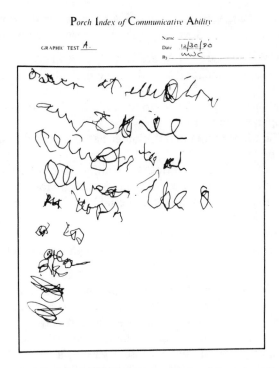

**Figure 8–5.** Patient's written description of PICA objects by function.

We were confronted, however, by a constellation of deficits, potential deficits, and nonlanguage characteristics that threatened to interfere with our goals. Some of these required direct management, some could be dealt with indirectly, some could be addressed simultaneously, and some could be handled sequentially. We established the following primary and immediate goals:

1. Stabilize yes-no responses to 80 to 90 percent correct, delayed responses (13s).
2. Improve gestural ability on 10 functional actions.
3. Improve writing ability to 10 functional words.
4. Reduce perseveration.
5. Reduce impulsivity.
6. Improve his ability to use a simplified communication board.

   The long-term goal was total communication. We believed our goal was realistic, given the patient's substantial deficits and his availability for treatment. We established a 1 hour, twice-daily treatment schedule that was the best compromise we could make among his other daily treatments, which would still give him time to rest.

Our treatment sessions followed a time-honored formula used by most clinicians in some form or other, and formalized by Porch (1981):

1. Adjustment period: "How are you?", general conversation, and so forth, with no demands placed on the patient and complete acceptance.
2. General activation: Warm-up period. Easy tasks, familiar tasks, fully operational tasks.
3. Consolidation: Old material. Somewhat more familiar tasks, not yet fully operational.
4. Modification: New material. Expanding task difficulty on a task now performed well—for example, from four foils to six foils.
5. Consolidation: Consolidate material worked on in the previous modification stage.
6. Modification: New material again.
7. Conclusion: Easy, familiar tasks, very high success rate.

Our first problem was finding an "easy" task to warm up on. We found one: Mr. Cross could sequence and match playing cards with few errors. The task served as a good introduction to treatment sessions in the early stages because the patient had been a card player, because the task seemed to be viewed as less a "task" than a game, because it allowed us to get Mr. Cross's attention, and because it gave us a task to begin building on. In our early sessions we also began to establish baselines for his "yes" and "no" responses to biographical questions, identification of body parts, and identification of pictured objects presented with one foil.

The "yes" and "no" questions were designed to be either highly salient ("Is your name Paul?") or highly disparate ("Is your name Angela Lansbury?"), and yes-no questions were presented alternately in the set of 10. He was allowed 5 to 10 seconds between each response, both to avoid "noise buildup" and to alert him to the end of one question and the beginning of another. Baseline performance averaged 20 percent, and this baseline was stable.

Identification of body parts is frequently better than performance on other tasks. Mr. Cross was an exception. He was unable to identify a single body part, although he followed some "axial" or whole body commands. This baseline was stable at 0 percent.

We selected 10 pictured, common objects from Marshall's program (1979). Baseline performance was again stable at 0 percent, and there was little variability in the type of response. The 2s reflect some ability to attend to the task, the 5s an intelligible response that was not related to the task, and the lonely 6 was an error—Mr. Cross pointed to the wrong object.

Treatment began tentatively, because Mr. Cross was sick and frequently irritable. We often had to limit our sessions to 30 minutes or even
less when he was less tolerant of us. Our treatment would eventually be
multifaceted, but in the beginning we concentrated on stabilizing the
"yes" and "no" responses, establishing the conditions both here and in
his hospital environment that would maximize input to him, treating his
auditory comprehension and his reading recognition skills, and trying to
get a foothold on a very basic, functional alternative mode of
communication.

We generally followed the protocol for stabilizing "yes" and "no"
responses. After a brief, introductory interlude, we introduced the next
module, presenting "yes" auditorily with Mr. Cross imitating the gesture
only. In the very early stages, we found it necessary to physically assist
him with the head nod. We were able to abandon that assistance after
four sessions. The first two sessions were limited to "yes." We would
ask a question, tell him the answer, and assist him with the gesture. If we
encountered resistance to our assistance, or the beginning of a movement
to a negative answer, we resisted, restated the answer, paused, and again
assisted him with the gesture. We introduced "time out" or "neutral"
after every response, and in this manner proceeded through 10 consecutive "yes" replies. By the third session the "yes" was nearly consistent
and reliable, and Mr. Cross no longer required physical assistance with
the response. We allowed one more session for stabilizing "yes" and
then began to introduce "no" in the same manner we had done with
"yes." "No" came more easily, and was consistent after two sessions.
We believed that we could begin to alternate the two responses, but very
cautiously and tentatively.

We began by presenting five questions that clearly required a "yes"
response, distinctly telling him we were about to begin another task, and
asking him five consecutive questions with "no" answers. Our criterion
for success at this point was 80 percent correct, but we did not tolerate
failure, and corrected and assisted the patient to make a correct
response.

We continued to test daily. We selected the morning sessions to probe,
because fatigue, particularly in the afternoon, had a significantly detri-
mental effect on Mr. Cross's performance. We also chose to probe at the
conclusion of treatment because at this point we were not as interested in
retention and carry-over. We wanted the patient to learn the task.

We believed that controlled auditory stimulation, to be effective,
requires a meaningful response to complete the circle, so our questions
to elicit "yes" and "no," therefore, were designed in part to maximize
auditory input as well as to elicit appropriate responses. We did not plan

to increase the complexity of our stimuli or reduce saliency or impact in the near future. We believed that the responses were too important to be left to the vicissitudes of stimulus complexity. Therefore, we tackled auditory comprehension on another front.

Using Marshall's *Clinician Controlled Auditory Stimulation,* we selected 10 common objects that could be succinctly identified by both name and function. We established baselines for pointing responses to these stimuli first by name and then by function. For the baseline task, each stimulus was presented with three foils. Baseline performance hovered near 10 percent but was somewhat variable. Again, because we were not expecting or looking for generalization, we planned a simple ABAB design (see Chapter 6).

We began our treatment of auditory comprehension with the first few steps of the playing card program. Performance was adequate and above chance expectations for the first few steps. We quickly reached asymptote, however, and although we continued to use the task as a warmup, only occasionally did we probe for success at higher levels.

Treatment, which began the next day and usually consumed about 15 minutes of each session, employed the first step of a somewhat modified natural language learning program. The target item, and only that item, was exposed until performance reached the 100 percent correct level. Our auditory stimulus during treatment was brief but redundant. We required a pointing response, with which we assisted him if necessary, and our stimuli contained both name and function for contextual redundancy (e.g., "Show me the broom. The one you sweep with"). As in previous tasks, we allowed for frequent exposures to silence, or "neutral," and clearly differentiated one task from the next. We reinforced the correct response, corrected an incorrect response, said something like "OK, that's it for that one," paused for approximately 5 seconds, then said something like "OK, here's the next one," and presented the stimulus.

When performance on probes of this task is compared with performance on object name and object function alone, it is apparent that contextual redundancy enhances Mr. Cross's comprehension. One of our goals was to share and reinforce that finding with staff members and family.

We used a similar technique to improve reading recognition. This task was preparatory to training in the use of an alternative communication system. When Mr. Cross could recognize, with reasonable consistency, 10 functional nouns that matched 10 pictures on a scaled-down version of the communication board (Fig. 8–6), we began to use the ability to enhance this aspect of his communicative process.

Mr. Cross's personal version also contained the name of each object or function in block letters, written immediately below each picture.

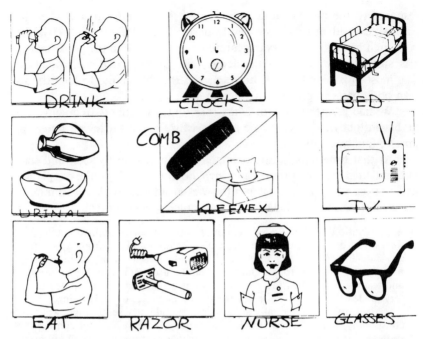

**Figure 8–6.** Individualized communication board for a globally aphasic patient. Developed by Mount Sinai Hospital of Cleveland, Ohio.   Cleo Living Aids, Cleveland, Ohio.

Again using a format similar to that for natural language learning, we concentrated on one picture at a time with no foils, presented stimuli with contextual redundancy, exposed another stimulus when appropriate, and retreated when it became obvious that we had exceeded the patient's capacity.

Performance in the early stages was variable, but the fluctuations were not extreme. We would have preferred greater fluctuations because we could then have modified our treatment accordingly. We placed few demands on auditory comprehension and fewer on selection, recall, and retrieval. We resisted the temptation to increase the difficulty of the stimuli, but we tested more difficult items occasionally just to remind ourselves to resist the temptation.

One final aspect of our treatment program focused on identification of body parts. We had found that only by chance was he correct in identifying even a single body part of his own, and he did no better when asked to identify body parts of others or from drawings. Because he could recognize photographs of other people with fair success, we believed that perhaps identifying body parts from a photograph would be more successful. We took a Polaroid picture of him, baselined his response to the picture, and compared these to performance when he was asked to identify his own body parts. The difference was striking. Although he was not always accurate on his first attempt, performance was significantly above chance levels, and he improved with practice. The most satisfying finding, however, was that his ability to identify his own body parts improved with treatment.

We had greater plans for Mr. Cross, but, as patients frequently do, he began lobbying to go home and, because he had a loving and supportive family, he did.

At that time he was approximately 2 months post onset, and serious, intensive rehabilitation, in which he could and would cooperate, had not lasted more than 1 month. We wrote our discharge summary regretfully, because we believed he had much greater potential:

> An evaluation of Mr. Cross's communicative abilities approximately 2 weeks post onset revealed a severe, global aphasia and no bright spots in any modality. Twice daily speech and language treatment began and continued until discharge today. Our treatment focused on improving auditory and reading comprehension and establishing an alternative or supplementary mode of communication for words and activities of daily living.
>
> Mr. Cross is still globally aphasic. He can identify some single words consistently, follows a few simple commands, copies a bit, and can even spontaneously write a few words. Spontaneous gestures are usually unintelligible and perseverative, however, but with assistance, repetition, and practice, a few gestures did improve. We were unsuccessful in getting him to use total communication—gestures have improved only minimally, he rejects most attempts at writing, and speech consists of brief, unintelligible utterances (with the exception of a few automatic phrases such as "forget it"), although "yes" and "no" are generally very clear. Perceptive abilities, however, have improved significantly. Performance on the LaPointe-Horner *Reading Comprehension Battery for Aphasia* improved from a mean of 2.7 correct to a mean of 5.6. Performance on the two auditory subtests of the *Porch Index of Communicative Ability* improved from a mean of 6.7 to 7.1, and Mr. Cross made modest gains in gestural ability. Speech and writing were unimproved. Overall performance on the PICA improved from the 10th to the 14th percentile. By any definition, Mr. Cross remains globally aphasic, and his prognosis for recovery of functional communicative skills is poor. Comprehension of speech and written material should continue to improve provided his physical condition does not deteriorate.
>
> We have agreed to see Mr. Cross twice weekly on an outpatient basis. Our goals are unchanged, but we will have less opportunity to implement our procedures and we suspect we will have to lower our sights unless he and his wife are compatible treatment partners and treatment can be extended to his home.
>
> We will reevaluate for progress in 3 months, which will be approximately 6 months post onset.

Mr. Cross continued to attend these twice weekly sessions for about a year. He attended regularly, in part because his wife brought him, in part because he seemed to enjoy the company and the chance to get out of the house, and in part because we think that he, and certainly his wife, recognized the gains he was making.

These gains, shown in Figure 8-7, show some improvement. Mr. Cross is still globally aphasic. Despite significant gains in writing, particularly copying ability, writing is not functional, and these skills have changed little over the years. A recent writing sample, taken at over 4 years post onset, is shown in Figure 8-8.

These sessions were directed toward solidifying the minimal gains Mr. Cross had made during his hospitalization, improving his ability to recall, identify, and write the names of his wife and children, and establish a core of useful, functional communications, predominantly written. Speech was still a potential channel, which he began to use more frequently to convey single words to represent longer messages, but his gestures were for the most part unintelligible, undifferentiated, and equivocal. "Yes" and "no" responses were now stable, although frequently they were incorrect if the questions were long, complex, or too

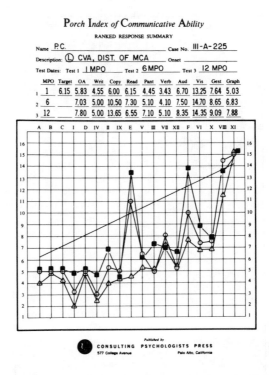

**Figure 8-7.** Graphic summary of performance on the PICA at 1, 6, and 12 months post onset.

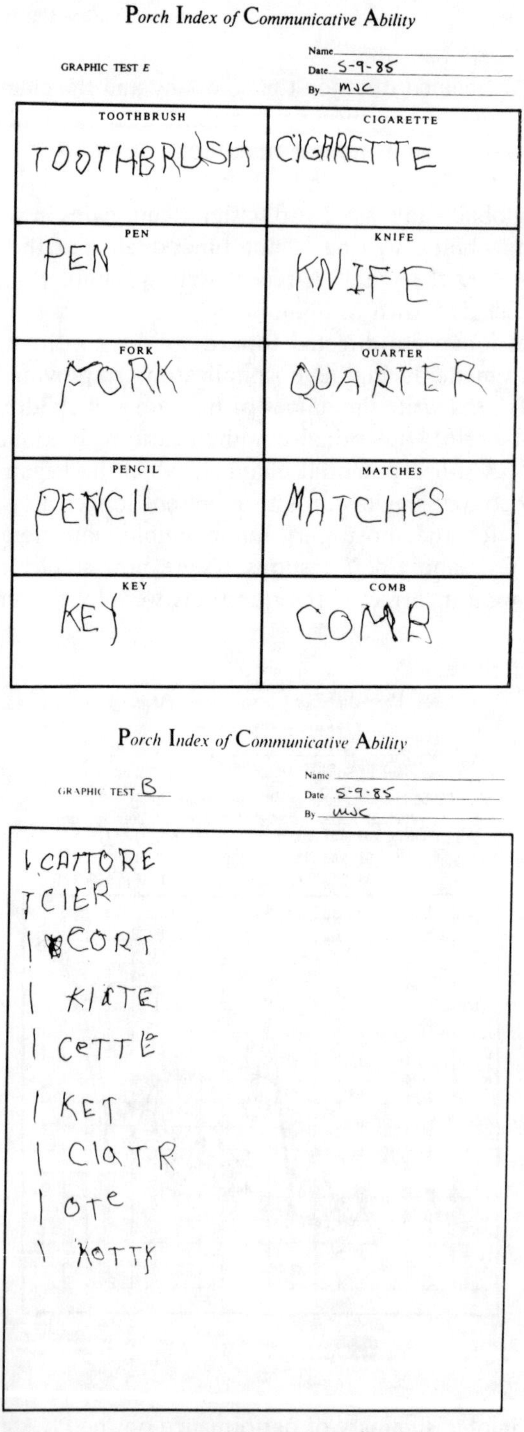
Porch Index of Communicative Ability

GRAPHIC TEST E

Name
Date 5-9-85
By MJC

| TOOTHBRUSH | CIGARETTE |
| --- | --- |
| TOOTHBRUSH | CIGARETTE |
| PEN | KNIFE |
| PEN | KNIFE |
| FORK | QUARTER |
| FORK | QUARTER |
| PENCIL | MATCHES |
| PENCIL | MATCHES |
| KEY | COMB |
| KEY | COMB |

Porch Index of Communicative Ability

GRAPHIC TEST B

Name
Date 5-9-85
By MJC

I CATTORE
I CIER
I CORT
I KIaTE
I CeTTE
I KET
I ClaTR
I OTe
I KOTTK

Figure 8–8. A recent writing sample from Mr. Cross.

fleeting. We continued to work on maintaining these gestures, but the need to do so became less and less pressing.

Mr. Cross's family was very important to him. They were involved in multifarious projects and activities and lived in different parts of the country. To help him keep track of them, we began a program that would allow him to identify them by name and by picture and to write their names, their occupations, and their addresses.

We obtained pictures of each family member from his wife. We made cards for each person, and separate cards with their occupation and hometown written on them. Our program followed the general procedures for writing and speech outlined in Chapter 6. More specific steps in this program, designed for this particular task and for Mr. Cross, are listed here.

Step  1.  Present single picture of family member with name alongside.
Step  2.  Say name three times, pausing for 3 seconds between each repetition.
Step  3.  Patient copies name twice.
Step  4.  Patient reads word, card is removed, patient writes name.
Step  5.  Clinician corrects or assists if necessary, says name.
Step  6.  Patient copies again.
Step  7.  Patient writes name after exposure of name card.
Step  8.  Patient writes name to dictation.
Step  9.  Clinician corrects if necessary, and Step 8 is repeated.
Step 10.  Patient repeats name.

Mr. Cross became successful at writing, and frequently at saying correctly, his wife's and each of his children's names. We were less successful at occupations and geographic locations. Mr. Cross uses a map successfully, and can frequently write a name and then tell us, by using the map, where a child is living or vacationing.

World-traveling children present more of a problem, and we never guessed that Peg in Luxembourg was really Mary in Venice, but we knew one of his children was in Europe.

We continue to see Mr. Cross on a regular basis, but much less frequently. He and his wife travel, and Mr. Cross attends a camp in northern Wisconsin for 2 weeks each summer. When he does see us, much of his time is spent on new gestures, reinforcing writing, and working on microcomputerized treatment programs.

These programs, all written for the Apple IIe with 64K RAM, are available commercially. Most have been designed to improve reading comprehension and spelling and are appropriate for many globally aphasic patients.

"Compu-Spell" is a program designed to improve spelling in context. There are six levels, corresponding approximately to readability or educational levels. Each level consists of 66 to 69 units, and each unit contains 10 sentences with a target word, usually a noun or verb, in each one. The target word is highlighted in each sentence initially. When the patient presses the space bar, the word is removed, and the patient is required to type in the word as he remembers it. Wrong letters are not accepted, but after several incorrect trials the word is spelled correctly for the patient.

Several factors in the program can be controlled and modified, including criterion level (10 to 100 percent), amount of context displayed in the posttest, and stimuli. Level 4, which includes predominantly common, monosyllabic words, is appropriate for many globally aphasic patients, as it is for Mr. Cross.

"Understanding Questions" is a program developed by Richard Katz (Sunset Software, 1983) which assesses and treats the ability to answer questions about who, what, why, where, and when. It too is appropriate for globally aphasic patients such as Mr. Cross, who retain, or have redeveloped, some ability to recognize words. The "who" and "what" questions are probably the simplest, and Mr. Cross now performs at approximately a 60 percent success level.

Another program that is suitable at some level for patients such as Mr. Cross, and can be adapted by the clinician to make it more suitable, is Apple's "Shell Games." One routine, a matching task, is especially suitable. As it is programmed, the learner is asked to match states to their capitals or animals to their collective nouns. This program itself is not especially useful except perhaps as entertainment or to acquaint the patient with the keyboard and the microcomputer. The programs can be adapted easily by the clinician, however, to make them more relevant to the patient.

For Mr. Cross, for example, we have been able to construct a program that allows him to match his children with their homes, the children with their occupations, and the occupations with the children.

There are undoubtedly other programs suitable for the globally aphasic patient. Many of these are listed in Chapter 7. The best of these programs, or the most useful, are those that allow clinicians who are computer novices to construct their own programs, as we have done for Mr. Cross.

Mr. Cross continues to improve, as our yearly testing demonstrates. He has exceeded his prognosis. His writing has improved significantly, as shown in Figure 8–8, but it is still functional only for family members' names and some other functional words, although his wife reports that he can often start a word, with the first letter, and by guessing she can understand the message.

Mr. Cross is blessed with a loving and patient wife who has more than endured the illness. She has accepted, helped, and questioned, and it has done him more good than all the therapy we have given him. She is honest and forthright, and she understands her husband's limitations. Mr. Cross is now 4 years post onset. We know he is better, and his test scores reveal some of that improvement. More of that improvement is revealed in his wife's rating of his functional communication abilities.

## GLOBAL APHASIA: IMPROVEMENT WITH ADJECTIVES

Mr. Richland was 56 years old when he suffered a massive left hemisphere CVA involving the frontal and temporal lobes. His major neurological residuals included a severe right hemiplegia, a right hemianesthesia, a right homonymous hemianopsia, and profound aphasia.

Our first evaluation, at bedside, took place at approximately 2 weeks post onset. Mr. Richland was ill, tired, and impatient with the staff members and their continual probes and needles as well as the endless stream of medical students. Our intrusion was not welcomed any more enthusiastically, and we began our evaluation covertly. We became passive observers of Mr. Richland's communicative interactions with staff members, family, and friends, and we infrequently penetrated his self-imposed barricades with a question or instruction. Our informal and subjective data told us that he was globally aphasic or nearly so. His "yes" and "no" responses were inappropriate and inconsistent, even to simple auditory stimuli. With the exception of a few automatic utterances ("goddam it" was his favorite), he was speechless. His dense hemiplegia was not confined to his limbs. He also displayed a pronounced right facial droop, and he was unable to control his saliva.

His prognosis for substantial recovery of speech and language skills was bleak. We did not share our pessimism with him or his family immediately, but we knew that this information would become critical when they began to plan their lives around his aphasia. Mr. Richland was the support and the foundation of a large family, and his aphasia would have a devastating effect on the family's financial and social futures. We did discuss the nature of aphasia and stroke with them, shared bibliographic materials, and supported and encouraged their attempts to communicate with him. They were provided with suggestions for communicating with the patient, and we tried to provide both a forum and an outlet for their frustrations and insecurities.

Two weeks after his stroke active rehabilitation began. His medical and neurological status had improved, and so had his attitude. These changes permitted us to form a more complete picture of his skills and deficits, but his tolerance for us and his frustration level were still low, and we continued to evaluate the patient more or less covertly. At 2 weeks post onset we arrived at the tentative conclusions reflected in our consultation report:

Mr. Richland was referred to us for evaluation of speech and language deficits following a left CVA 11-16-80. Informal observation and formal testing reveal the following:

*Listening:* Listening is severely impaired. Mr. Richland usually is unable to follow even simple instructions unless they are accompanied by gestures or appropriate pointing to objects or persons. He does follow a number of whole body commands fairly consistently. He moves his wheelchair when requested, and he glances at his watch when asked the time. He cannot be expected to remember or follow instructions or commands involving more than one step, and those commands must be repeated and reinforced. His communicative skills are not yet functional or independent, and care should be taken not to place too many demands on him; in addition he should not be expected to remember and follow instructions to take his medications or go to appointments independently.

Mr. Richland's auditory skills are improving and he is able to identify correctly single words presented auditorily about 50 percent of the time. These deficits are compounded by a severe binaural hearing loss, which was present premorbidly. He was a reasonably good candidate for a hearing aid before the CVA and, although he is not as good a candidate now, when he has improved sufficiently to be helped by the device we would recommend one.

*Reading:* Reading is severely impaired. Mr. Richland is able to recognize single words at a level slightly above chance, but he is unable to make associations among printed stimuli and objects or pictures.

*Writing:* Writing is impossible to assess at this time because the patient has rejected all attempts to test writing or copying ability. It is probable that writing ability is as impaired as speaking.

*Speech:* Speech is severely impaired. His speech consists of several recurring utterances, such as "I never," "goddam it," and "Well, I don't know." The phrases are automatic, and are appropriate only by chance. His deficits in speech production are not due to weakness or paralysis despite his right lower facial weakness. He has a severe oral, nonverbal apraxia and probably a severe apraxia of speech.

*Impressions:* Severe, global aphasia. Mr. Richland's ability to use language will improve, but it is too early to tell how much improvement to expect. The extent and location of his lesion suggest that the evolution of his aphasia, if it occurs, will be from global aphasia to what Mohr et al. (1978) called a "big" Broca aphasia, in which speech is telegraphic, halting, awkwardly articulated, and dysgrammatic. The patient's prognosis is improved by his relative youth, the recency of onset of the disorder, his premorbid occupational and educational attainment, and the existence of a strong, supportive family who will support, encourage, and stimulate him. His severe hearing loss and coexisting medical problems (hypertension and diabetes) are not in his favor. If he is to regain functional communication skills, treatment must be intense and protracted.

We will see this patient at least twice daily during the course of his hospitalization and make periodic reevaluations of his progress. We have begun counseling his family to explain the nature of his deficits and to guide them in their efforts to communicate with him.

## Early Evaluation and Treatment

Mr. Richland's fragile psyche dictated that initial treatment sessions be brief. We placed limited demands on him to perform specific tasks. We began by assessing his ability to respond to questions and to follow simple commands using whole body and axial movements. These included questions such as, "Can you tell me the time?" "What does the weather look like?" He could follow these and many other questions and commands when presented in a conversational context or when they involved body parts. He could take his glasses off on command, open and close his eyes, and make a fist. Efforts to prompt him to attempt more structured treatment tasks led to failure, frustration, and rejection, and eventually even those benign attempts took a toll. Mr. Richland rejected our services and refused to come to treatment.

Three days later he voluntarily (with the encouragement of his wife and family) returned to the clinic, but on his own terms. He was unwilling to do anything he perceived as treatment or testing, but he appeared to enjoy whatever interactions he had with us, especially when we received one of his messages accurately.

At 6 weeks post onset, our approach had yielded some dividends. Mr. Richland was still severely aphasic, but by this time he was showing some promise that he would move out of the global aphasia range. The variety and frequency of real words he could use had increased, consisting almost entirely of nouns and verbs or approximations of them. His auditory comprehension, reading, and writing had improved, and he could now follow some complex commands, identify, repeat, copy, and read a few single words aloud, and could play a few card games like poker and blackjack.

Our early intervention was designed to stimulate, facilitate, and elicit as much diagnostic and treatment information as we could and to provide unobtrusive treatment that was appropriate, that he could do with a high degree of success, and that he was willing to do. This might be called therapy by default, but that did not make the treatment any less valuable or necessary. We persevered because we recognized the patient's potential, because his family wanted treatment, and because in the early stages of treatment Mr. Richland was not physically or emotionally ready for treatment or to make an informed choice. He was anxious to leave the hospital at approximately 3 months post onset. He was walking, with the assistance of a cane, but he was not talking much. Three weeks later his wife asked us to see him as an outpatient, and we agreed to a 60 day trial period.

We administered the *Porch Index of Communicative Ability* at 4 months post onset. The test was difficult for the patient and required nearly 70 minutes to administer. His overall score was 8.66, which placed him at the 28th percentile for aphasic adults. He rejected all writing tasks, but performance was somewhat better on copying tasks. An example, PICA subtest E, is shown in Figure 8–9.

Using Porch's HOAP slopes, we projected performance to the 43rd percentile at 6 months post onset, but that optimistic projection was tempered somewhat by his poor performance on tasks that did not require imitation, copying, or gesturing.

A test for oral nonverbal and limb apraxia revealed significant deficits, although almost without exception performance improved with practice and instruction. Performance on the *Coloured Progressive Matrices* was 24 correct, which placed him between the 40th and 50th percentile for aphasic adults, another optimistic finding. Finally, we administered the *Boston Diagnostic Aphasia Examination*. A subjective rating of the severity of his aphasia was 1, and the rating scale profile of speech characteristics was typical of that seen in very severe Broca's aphasia.

## Treatment Planning

Because Mr. Richland's performance profile seemed somewhat atypical, we constructed an individualized Ranked Response Summary for him. His performance curve was variable and atypical, as shown in Figure 8–10. It suggests a clear progression of difficulty for him. It corresponds only generally to the typical Ranked Response Summary. From this profile, we selected several tasks, which the patient performed relatively well, and which promised to be succeeded by better performance on more difficult tasks. Mr. Richland did not share our enthusiasm for these treatment targets. He resisted all therapeutic endeavors that did not involve speech. We knew, and perhaps he knew as well, that we might struggle for years and never achieve that goal. We tried to help him recognize that other forms of communication were valuable, too, but we also wanted him to know that because we did not work on speech exclusively did not mean that we were not optimistic. Because speaking meant so much to him, speech drill became a part of his program. We encouraged speech, and applauded his successes, but gave speech a secondary role in treatment.

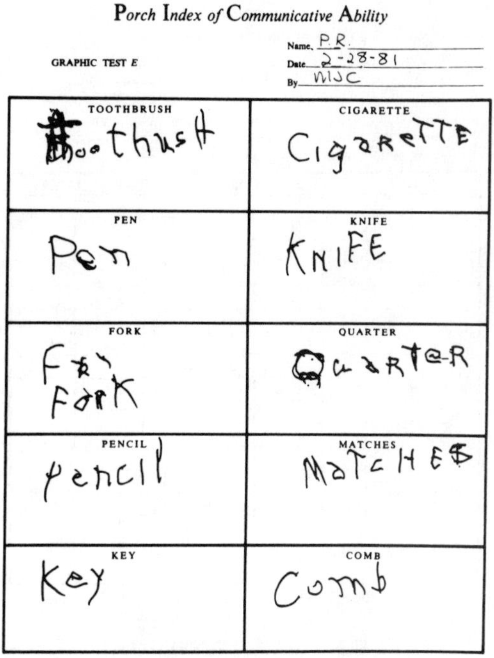

Porch Index of Communicative Ability

GRAPHIC TEST E

Name PR.
Date 2-28-81
By WJC

**Figure 8–9.** PICA subtest E.

Initially his "yes" and "no" responses were ambiguous and equivocal. He often said "yes" when he meant "no" or gestured "yes" and
said "no." His failure only increased his frustration, and that of his
listeners. We began our treatment by having him point to cards labeled
"yes" and "no," and despite his resistance we insisted that pointing to
either of those cards was the only response we would accept. We also
assured him that this stage was only temporary. We acknowledged every
response and corrected his mistakes, and we insisted that every stimulus
and each response have a consequence. Questions were simple and direct
and as salient as possible. Because his responses, and his reading comprehension, were better than Mr. Cross's, we began with several brief
sessions, drilling first "yes," then "no," and then began to alternate
"yes" and "no" in answer to a series of biographical questions. When
we thought the response was stable, we began to pair gestural responses
with pointing to "yes" and "no" cards. In this stage, which lasted only
a few sessions, Mr. Richland was asked to respond to the same questions
asked in the earlier stage, but he was required to first point to the correct
word and then gesture "yes" by nodding his head or "no" by shaking
his head. We continued to inhibit verbal responses because they were so
unstable, but it was clear that in this patient gestural and pointing

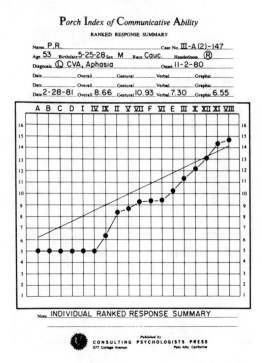

Figure 8–10. Graphic representation of performance on the 18 PICA subtests (in order of difficulty) by Mr. Richland.

responses would eventually yield to verbal responses. We began to pair the gestural responses with verbal responses, in a drill that simulated gestural reorganization. "Yes" and "no" had always been intelligible, so our goal was not to elicit these replies but to elicit them when they were appropriate. Two sessions were required to stabilize the paired responses to the previously baselined questions. The stability of this response suggested that it was safe to fade the gestural response, but we encouraged Mr. Richland to use it if he felt uncertain or unsure of his response. His reliance on gestures gradually faded, but we continued to caution him to pause, be sure of his response, and then respond.

## Gesturing

In early sessions, we assessed spontaneous gestural ability informally in conversation, formally in response to pictured or auditory stimuli, and imitatively. Intact gestures were incorporated into a corpus of gestures to be trained in therapy. Ten gesturable actions (for example, eat, drink, walk, and listen) were selected for practice. When the patient could not pantomime the desired response, we used real objects. When all gestures could be elicited on command, pantomime training began. Beginning with one gesture, we presented both spoken and gestured stimuli until that gesture was intact. We encouraged, but did not force, verbal imitation to accompany the gesture. When that gesture was intact, regardless of whether verbalization accompanied it, we expanded to two gestures, alternating between the two, with fewer repetitions of each until Mr. Richland could alternate gestures successively through the final step. As he progressed, we added gestures and repeated the process until all three gestures were firmly established. A Base-10 showing his response to that program is given in Figure 8–11.

Once he had learned several gestures, used them in response to questions, and, we hoped, recognized the need for them, they were incorporated into a program of total communication. Pointing was an integral part of that program and was used to convey a primary message as well as to impart attributes of an object or concept. We incorporated contextual pointing in a program of total communication by first establishing a clear, unequivocal gesture. Initially, the accuracy of the response was not nearly so important as establishing a clear response. We asked Mr. Rich-

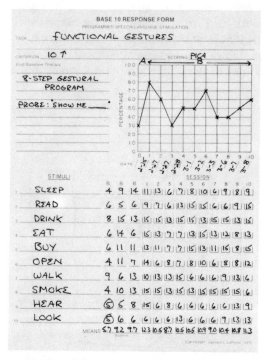

**Figure 8–11.** Graphic representation of performance on a gestural program, AB design.

land to point to one object, or pictured object, with no foil. When the response was inadequate, we had him imitate the gesture until it was intact. As response adequacy increased, we added one foil and drilled each step until adequacy was achieved. Next, the stimulus field was expanded by asking the patient to point to objects in the room, imitating our gestures when necessary. In the final stage, he was asked to look at a series of realistic colored pictures, first pointing to objects we identified, then pointing to corresponding items in the room. We used a similar procedure for conveying attributes such as color by having him point to objects of the same color as the target.

## Drawing

Perhaps because sketching and diagramming had been so important in his work, Mr. Richland retained an ability to draw a few simple pictures. We decided to capitalize on that ability. Much of his leisure time was spent on his farm, where despite his hemiplegia he had begun again to tend to the horses, the fences, and the lawn. We asked him to draw a diagram of his property. His first attempt, shown in Figure 8–12, improved in a few weeks to the attempt shown in Figure 8–13. Several months later, with help from his wife and his clinician, he produced the result shown in Figure 8–14, reduced in size from 16 by 20 inches. We encouraged him to practice drawing at home and enlisted his wife's help. We also asked him to draw diagrams of his house and hometown and

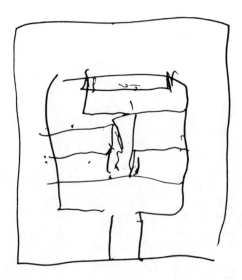

**Figure 8–12.**  Initial attempt by Mr. Richland to diagram his property.

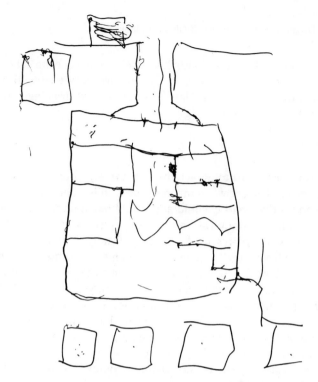

**Figure 8–13.** Second attempt by Mr. Richland to diagram his property.

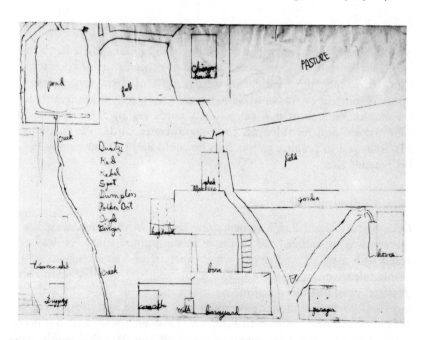

**Figure 8–14.** Most recent attempt by Mr. Richland to diagram his property.

frequently traveled routes. With his wife's assistance he labeled these drawings and brought them to the clinic, where we embellished, corrected, and drilled him in the labels, legends, and drawings, and tested him with them periodically.

## Writing

Writing is a time-consuming activity for severely aphasic patients and is probably most efficient when much of the drill is done outside the clinic. We felt certain that writing could and would be an important part of Mr. Richland's total communication program. Initially, we selected 40 functional words which represented activities of daily living, words that were salient and relevant for him, including names of family members. We baselined these words for three sessions, and then four word lists were selected and equated for difficulty. We employed an ABAB design in which the treatment was copying drill at home followed by copying with assistance, feedback, and reinforcement in the clinic. We could not control the amount of time he spent in copying practice at home. He practiced as much as he could find time for, and we sacrificed some part of our internal validity. The results of that program, in Base-10 form, are shown in Figure 8-15.

## Speech

Mr. Richland's relatively good repetition skill made it difficult to resist the temptation to work on speech instead of other forms of communication. He worked on a variety of words, most of them very salient for him. We thought he was unlikely to practice his errors at home, provided the stimuli were short and salient. All words assigned for speech drill were written and recorded on Language Master cards. We encouraged Mr. Richland to practice as much as he could and to keep a daily log of his practice time.

## Total Communication

Once Mr. Richland had regained some facility in each modality, PACE therapy was introduced. To facilitate this communication, he was provided with a pencil and paper, which were treated as extensions of the communicative process. Initially, using realistic colored cards that depicted only one clear action, we asked him to describe the action in any or all of the communicative modalities open to him. Responses that communicated the action were accepted. These responses were not necessarily accurate, but they communicated. When Mr. Richland's reply

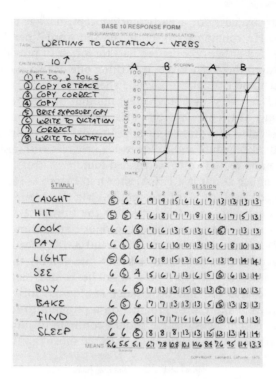

**Figure 8–15.** Graphic representation of performance on a writing program, ABAB design.

communicated, our response was a modeling of his response. When he failed to communicate, we modeled an acceptable model for him to imitate. As competence improved, the patient's vocabulary core was expanded, and when he could communicate approximately 10 of these actions, we began exchanges in more natural communicative topics. The clinician and Mr. Richland alternated as speaker and listener. As the patient's ability improved we began to incorporate his activities and interests in this paradigm and involved his family, particularly his wife, in the treatment. The themes involved his family, hobbies, travel, and current events. In our clinic sessions, we asked him to identify one or two themes for discussion, or we selected a theme. As a theme was developed, central and related descriptors were added. In these early sessions most of the burden of communication was on the clinician.

In subsequent sessions we transferred as much of the burden of communication to Mr. Richland as he would accept. He became adept at communicating in a variety of "languages," even though only part of a message was contained in each modality; if one modality did not provide him with any avenues for a particular concept, he was not reluctant to try another. He spontaneously produced the word "pen" or "paper" when he needed either or when we had forgotten to provide the materials, and he used them effectively by writing one or two expressive words.

Mr. Richland's treatment became sporadic after the first year. With his physical recovery and a greater amount of leisure time he had resumed many of his previous activities, although his hemiplegia and his aphasia prevented him from returning to work. We obliged in allowing an intermittent schedule and followed his progress with testing when we could. When he requested it, we treated him.

Performance at our last PICA, shown in Figure 8-16, never reached the predicted level of 43rd percentile. Mr. Richland's writing has improved somewhat, and it is better for the things he knows best. He does not produce sentences but can produce approximations of many single words, as shown in Figures 8-17 and 8-18. Because he is such a tenacious achiever, we believe he is better functionally than his test performance shows. At 5 years post onset he is still making gains. He recently discovered our microcomputer and comes in more frequently. He is presently making slow progress on a program to improve spelling and reading comprehension. He should continue to improve, although these gains may not be striking except to the most careful observer.

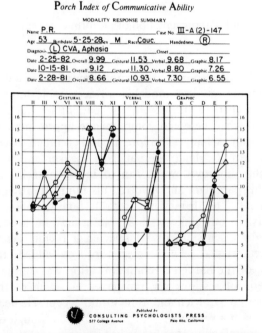

Figure 8-16. Graphic representation, by modality, of PICA performance at 4 months, 1 year, and 16 months post onset.

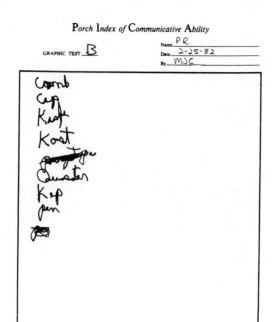

**Figure 8–17.** Approximations of single words written by Mr. Richland at time of his last PICA.

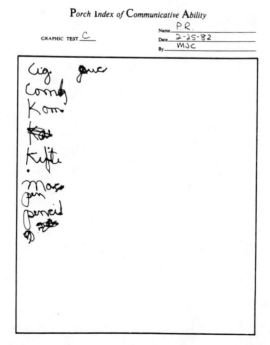

**Figure 8–18.** Approximations of single words written by Mr. Richland at time of his last PICA.

# Epilogue

This book began with a tentative definition of global aphasia, which may not stand the test of time but will serve our purposes for the present. This definition represents an attempt to synthesize what we have learned about global aphasia. The most important feature of the definition, perhaps, is that it suggests that global aphasia is common in early stages of recovery from cerebral lesions but invariably it evolves.

The chapters that followed represent an attempt to merge what is known about global aphasia with what is known about treatment and its effects on recovery. A brief summary of the reasonably solid evidence suggests that global aphasia generally results from large cortical lesions of the left hemisphere; that global aphasia is dynamic and frequently evolves into a less severe form; that a substantial number of patients do not recover from the global deficits; and that nonlinguistic sequelae generally are more severe as magnitude of the lesion increases. The evidence also suggests that recovery patterns in global aphasia differ from those seen in other types of aphasia: frequently recovery accelerates in the later stages of recovery, and this recovery may be related to physiological factors.

The right hemisphere played a prominent role in the discussion because it holds such promise for reacquisition of language. The evidence cited here suggests that this substantial promise is still probably just that, perhaps because we have not learned to capitalize on this potential, or perhaps because it is more promise than substance.

Diagnosis and treatment are both highlighted because the author believes that the best treatment cannot proceed without the best evaluation. Both formal and informal testing play a legitimate role in evaluation, but informal testing should play a subordinate role to formal testing, at least until the data bases and standardization of both types of testing are equated.

The argument is raised here that the prediction of eventual recovery levels, although still an imprecise science, is more important to families and to treatment planning than it is to clinicians' egos. With the knowledge that aphasia will evolve, we can within certain broad limits quantify and make predictions about this evolution. That prediction is imprecise is less a comment on our primitive methods than it is on intangible attributes of spirit and character.

Darley (1982) says that "the bulk of the data from all the studies would compel one to believe that no single factor that negatively influences recovery appears to be so uniformly potent as to justify automatically excluding a patient from at least a trial of therapy on the basis of its existence" (p. 183). The negative factors Darley means include severity of aphasia. A number of treatment techniques exist that promise to enhance significantly the quality of communication for the globally aphasic patient. These techniques are most effective when the aphasia is fresh, the deficits are yielding, and the aphasia is destined to evolve. It is not known which of the techniques is most efficacious under the conditions just described because they have not been adequately tested. A limited number of techniques, however, may have more robust effects on chronic, enduring global aphasia, even that which in time becomes very severe aphasia of a distinct subtype. These include gestural training, VAT, PACE, and Total Communication. Other promising techniques include Natural Language Learning, VCIU, and artificial language training. All of these methods merit further study. Clinicians, whose business is treating, should also make it their business to think about how best to improve their techniques. As this book implies, there is indeed much to think about.

# Appendix

## RATING OF FUNCTIONAL PERFORMANCE

Patient Name: _____

Date Form Completed: _____

Person Completing Form: _____

Relationship to Patient: _____

1. Cannot do what is asked in the question.
2. Usually cannot do what is asked in the question, but patient has done it infrequently since the stroke.
3. Can do what is asked in the question about half of the time, but the other half of the time patient cannot.
4. Patient can do what is asked in the question most of the time, but every now and then he or she cannot or makes mistakes.
5. No difficulty doing what is asked in the question and can do it as well as people who have not had a stroke.

Recognition or Understanding
1. Responds to adversive stimuli (e.g., threat, danger, angry voice tone, etc.).
2. Responds to sounds around the house.
3. Responds to his own name.
4. Aware of speech (e.g., looks at you when you talk to him, looks from person to person when several people are talking)?
5. Recognizes family names?
6. Understands single words (e.g., door, paper, look, walk)?
7. Understands short phrases (e.g., pass the salt, open the window)?

8. Appears to understand simple conversation with one person and responds appropriately?
9. Watches TV or listens to radio and responds appropriately (e.g., laughs at the right time, hums or taps foot to music)?
10. Aware of emotional voice tone?
11. Understands gestured directions?
12. Benefits from multimodal instructions (e.g., gesture with speech, written with speech)?
13. Learns simple task sequences (e.g., operating a calculator, using a Language Master)?
14. Learns or demonstrates inherent ability to play simple card games (e.g., "21," gin rummy, solitaire)?
15. Learns and follows a daily schedule?
16. Has at least a basic comprehension of monetary relationships (e.g., making change)?
17. Performs simple household chores?

(Clinician will complete)   Mean Score _____

Responding
1. Unequivocal "yes" "no" responses.
2. Often gestures appropriately.
3. Demonstrates simple sequenced activities.

(Clinician will complete)   Mean Score _____

Reading
1. Recognizes pictures (e.g., of family members).
2. Recognizes his name.
3. Reads and understands traffic and street signs.
4. Reads and understands individual letters of the alphabet.
5. Reads and understands single words (e.g., boat, work, lunch).
6. Uses telephone book or other common resource material.
7. Reads and understands short phrases (e.g., take out the garbage, back at 12:00).
8. Reads and understands newspaper headlines.
9. Reads and understands letters from family members and friends.
10. Reads and understands newspaper stories and magazine articles.
11. Reads and understands complicated directions (e.g., for filling out a form, for putting a toy together).

(Clinician will complete)   Mean Score _____

Speaking
1. Social greetings (e.g., hello, good-bye, thank you)?
2. Says "yes" and "no" appropriately?
3. Says single words appropriately (e.g., hot, early, milk)?
4. Says two-word phrases appropriately (e.g.,"home Saturday," 'my wife," "too hard")?
5. Says short phrases appropriately (e.g., "be here tomorrow?," "I can't do it")?
6. Asks for directions?

7. Says short sentences appropriately (e.g., "I want some milk," "My throat hurt," "Bring me the paper")?
8. Says long, complex sentences appropriately?

(Clinician will complete)   Mean Score _____

Writing
1. Draws recognizable shapes or pictures.
2. Copies the letters of the alphabet.
3. Writes or prints the letters of the alphabet without seeing a model.
4. Writes his name.
5. Writes or prints words if someone spells them for him.
6. Writes or prints single words on his own.
7. Writes or prints short phrases on his own (e.g., come back, a glass of milk).
8. Writes or prints complete sentences.
9. Writes or prints notes or make lists.
10. Writes or prints letters to family or friends.

(Clinician will complete)   Mean Score _____

Other
1. Can he convey his wants by gesturing (e.g., pointing, shaking his head, sounds)?
2. Can he take care of his basic needs by himself (eating, bathroom, dressing)?
3. Does he know where he is at all times (e.g., city, state, home hospital)?
4. Can he keep track of time (e.g., keep appointments, on time for meals, knows when TV programs are on)?
5. Can he play simple games (e.g., checkers, cards, bingo)?
6. Can he do simple household chores (e.g., gardening, dishes, cleaning)?
7. Can he get to speech therapy by himself (e.g., walk, wheelchair, taxi, bus, drive)?
8. Can he do errands in the neighborhood (e.g., pick up items from store, return items to neighbors, mail letters)?
9. Can he use money appropriately (e.g., purchase items, pay the correct amount, make change)?
10. Can he do arithmetic (e.g., add, subtract, multiply, and divide)?

(Clinician will complete)   Mean Score _____

(Clinician will complete)   OVERALL MEAN _____

# REFERENCES

Alajouanine, T., and Lhermitte, F. (1960). Les troubles des activities expressives du langage dans l'aphasie et leurs relations avec les apraxias. *Revue Neurologique, 102,* 604–629.

Archer, L. (1977). Blissymbolics—a nonverbal communication system. *Journal of Speech and Hearing Disorders, 42,* 568–579.

Asher, J. (1981). Fear of foreign language. *Psychology Today, 15,* 52–56.

Aten, J., Kushner-Vogel, D., Haire, A., West, J.F., O'Connor, S., and Bennet, L. (1981). Group treatment for aphasia: A panel discussion. In R. Brookshire (Ed.), *Proceedings of the conference on clinical aphasiology.* Minneapolis: BRK Publishers.

Aten, J.L., Caligiuri, M.P., and Holland, A.L. (1982). The efficacy of functional communication therapy for chronic aphasic patients. *Journal of Speech and Hearing Disorders, 47,* 93–96.

Bailey, S. (1978). Blissymbolics for dysphasics: A case report. *Blissymbolics Communication Institute Newsletter, 5,* 18–22.

Bales, R.F. (1970). *Personality and interpersonal behavior.* New York: Holt, Rinehart and Winston.

Benson, D.F. (1979). *Aphasia, alexia, and agraphia.* New York: Churchill Livingstone, Inc.

Boller, F., and Green, E. (1972). Comprehension in severe aphasia. *Cortex, 8,* 382–394.

Bollinger, R.L., and Stout, C.E. (1974). Response contingent small step treatment. In R. Brookshire (Ed.), *Proceedings of the conference on clinical aphasiology.* Minneapolis: BRK Publishers.

Boone, D. (1965). *An adult has aphasia.* Danville, IL: The Interstate Printers and Publishers, Inc.

Broida, H. (1977). Language therapy effects in long term aphasia. *Archives of Physical Medicine and Rehabilitation, 58,* 238–253.

Carson, D.H., Carson, F.E., and Tikofsky, R.S. (1968). On learning characteristics of the adult aphasic. *Cortex, 4,* 92–112.

Chapey, R. (1981). Divergent semantic intervention. In R. Chapey (Ed.), *Language intervention strategies in adult aphasia.* Baltimore: Williams and Wilkins.

Cohen, W.J. (1968, December 28). Letter to the Honorable John W. McCormack transmitting HEW report on the "Independent Practitioners Study."

Colby, K., Christinaz, D., Parkison, R., Graham, S., and Karpf, C. (1981). A word-finding computer program with a dynamic lexical-semantic memory for patients with anomia using an intelligent speech prosthesis. *Brain and Language, 14,* 272–281.

Collins, M.J. (1982). Unpublished data.

Collins, M.J., and Wertz, R.T. (1983). Coping with success: The maintenance of therapeutic effect in aphasia. In R. Brookshire (Ed.), *Proceedings of the conference on clinical aphasiology.* Minneapolis: BRK Publishers.

Collins, M.J., and Wertz, R.T. (1974). Classical conditioning in aphasic adults. In B. Porch (Ed.), *Proceedings of the Conference on Clinical Aphasiology.* Albuquerque: Veterans Administration Hospital.

Conniff, R. (1983). Prisoners without a language. *Dial, 4,* 38–39.

Darley, F.L. (1976). Maximizing input to the aphasic patient: A review of the literature. In R. Brookshire (Ed.), *Proceedings of the conference on clinical aphasiology.* Minneapolis: BRK Publishers.

Darley, F.L. (1979). Treat or neglect? *ASHA, 21,* 628–631.

Darley, F.L. (1982). *Aphasia.* Philadelphia: W.B. Saunders Co.

Davis, G.A. (1982). *A survey of adult aphasia.* Englewood Cliffs, NJ: Prentice-Hall.

Davis, G.A., and Wilcox, M.J. (1981). Incorporating parameters of natural conversation in aphasia treatment. In R. Chapey (Ed.), *Language intervention strategies in adult aphasia.* Baltimore: Williams and Wilkins.

Davis, G.A., and Wilcox, M.J. (1985). *Adult aphasia rehabilitation: applied pragmatics.* San Diego: College-Hill Press.

deBleser, R., and Poeck, K. (1983, October). *Analysis of prosody in the spontaneous speech of patients with CV-recurring utterances.* Paper presented at the Academy of Aphasia Meeting, Minneapolis.

de Bleser, R., and Poeck, K. (1984). Aphasia with exclusively consonant-vowel recurring utterances: Tan-Tan revisited. In F.C. Rose (Ed.), *Advances in neurology, Vol. 42: Progress in aphasiology.* New York: Raven Press.

Dennis, M. (1980). Capacity and strategy for syntactic comprehension after left or right hemidecortication. *Brain and Language, 10,* 287–317.

DeRenzi, E., and Vignolo, L.A. (1962). The token test: A sensitive test to detect receptive disturbances in aphasia. *Brain, 85,* 665–678.

Duffy, J.R. (1979). Review of the *Boston Diagnostic Aphasia Examination.* In F.L. Darley (Ed.), *Evaluation of appraisal techniques in speech and language pathology.* Reading, MA: Addison-Wesley Publishing Company.

Duffy, J.R. (1981). Schuell's stimulation approach to rehabilitation. In R. Chapey (Ed.), *Language intervention strategies in adult aphasia.* Baltimore: Williams and Wilkins.

Edelman, G.M. (1984). Assessment of understanding in global aphasia. In F.C. Rose (Ed.), *Advances in neurology: Progress in aphasiology.* New York: Raven Press.

Fromm, D., Holland, A.L., and Swindell, C.S. (1984). Depression following left hemisphere stroke (abstract). In R. Brookshire (Ed.), *Proceedings of the conference on clinical aphasiology.* Minneapolis: BRK Publishers.

Gardner, H., Zurif, E.B., Berry, T., and Baker, E. (1976). Visual communication in aphasia. *Neuropsychologia, 14,* 95–103.

Gazzaniga, M.E. (1971). Language and speech capacity of the right hemisphere. *Neuropsychologia, 9,* 273–280.

Geschwind, N., and Levitsky, W. (1968). Human brain: Left-right asymmetries in temporal speech region. *Science, 161,* 186–187.

Glass, A.V., Gazzaniga, M., and Premack, D. (1973). Artificial language training in global aphasics. *Neuropsychologica, 11,* 95–103.

Goda, S. (1962). Spontaneous speech, an primary source of therapy material. *Journal of Speech and Hearing Disorders, 27,* 190–192.

Goodglass, H. (1981). The syndromes of aphasia: Similarities and differences in neurolinguistic features. *Topics in Language Disorders, 1,* 1–14.

Goodglass, H., and Kaplan, E. (1963). Disturbance of gesture and pantomime in aphasia. *Brain, 86,* 703–720.

Goodglass, H., and Kaplan, E. (1972, 1983). *The assessment of aphasia and related disorders.* Philadelphia: Lea and Febiger.

Gray, L., Hoyt, P., Mogil, S., and Lefkowitz, N. (1977). A comparison of clinical tests of yes/no questions in aphasia. In R. Brookshire (Ed.), *Proceedings of the conference on clinical aphasiology.* Minneapolis: BRK Publishers.

Green, E., and Boller, F. (1974). Features of auditory comprehension in severely impaired aphasics. *Cortex, 10,* 133–146.

Haskins, S. (1976). A treatment procedure for writing disorders. In R. Brookshire (Ed.), *Proceedings of the conference on clinical aphasiology.* Minneapolis: BRK Publishers.

Held, J.P. (1975). The natural history of stroke. In S. Licht (Ed.), *Stroke and its rehabilitation.* Baltimore: Waverly Press.

Helm, N., and Barresi, B. (1980). Voluntary control of involuntary utterances: A treatment approach for severe aphasia. In R. Brookshire (Ed.), *Proceedings of the conference on clinical aphasiology.* Minneapolis: BRK Publishers.

Helm, N., and Benson, F. (1978). *Visual action therapy for global aphasia.* Paper presented at the Academy of Aphasia, Chicago.

Helm-Estabrooks, N.A. (1981). "Show me the ————— whatever": Some variables affecting auditory comprehension scores of aphasic patients. In R. Brookshire (Ed.), *Proceedings of the conference on clinical aphasiology.* Minneapolis: BRK Publishers.

Helm-Estabrooks, N., Fitzpatrick, P.M., and Barresi, B. (1982). Visual action therapy for global aphasia. *Journal of Speech and Hearing Disorders, 47,* 385–389.

Helm-Estabrooks, N., and Walsh, M. (1982). *Response of aphasic patients to an electronic communication board.* Paper presented at the Annual Convention of the American Speech-Language-Hearing Association, Toronto, Canada.

Hillinger, M., Fox, B., and Wilson, M. (1981). Computer-enhanced communication systems for the Apple II. In *Proceedings of the Johns Hopkins First Annual Search for Applications of Personal Computing to Aid the Handicapped.* Los Angeles: IEEE Computing Society.

Holland, A. (1970). Case studies in aphasia rehabilitation using programmed instruction. *Journal of Speech and Hearing Disorders, 35* (4), 371–390.

Holland, A. (1977). Some practical considerations in aphasia rehabilitation. In M. Sullivan and M.S. Kommers (Eds.), *Rationale for adult aphasia therapy*. Omaha: University of Nebraska Medical Center.

Holland, A. (1980). *Communicative abilities in daily living*. Baltimore: University Park Press.

Holland, A. (1982). Observing functional communication of aphasic adults. *Journal of Speech and Hearing Disorders. 47,* 50–56.

Holland, A. (1983). Remarks on observing aphasic people. In R. Brookshire (Ed.), *Proceedings of the conference on clinical aphasiology*. Minneapolis: BRK Publishers.

Horner, J., and LaPointe, L.L. (1979). Evaluation of learning potential of a severe aphasic adult through analysis of five performance variables. In R. Brookshire (Ed.), *Proceedings of the conference on clinical aphasiology*. Minneapolis: BRK Publishers.

Houghton, P.M., Pettit, J.M., and Towey, M.P. (1982). Measuring Communication Competence in global aphasia. In R. Brookshire (Ed.), *Proceedings of the conference on clinical aphasiology*. Minneapolis: BRK Publishers.

Jaynes, J. (1976). *The origin of consciousness in the breakdown of the bicameral mind*. Boston: Houghton Mifflin.

Johannsen-Horbach, H., Cegla, B., Mager, U., Schempp, B., and Wallesch, C. (1985). Treatment of chronic global aphasia with a nonverbal communication system. *Brain and Language, 24,* 74–82.

Katz, R. (1983). *Understanding Questions* (computer program). Los Angeles: Sunset Software, Inc.

Katz, R., and Tong-Nagy, V. (1982). A computerized treatment system for chronic aphasic patients. In R. Brookshire (Ed.), *Proceedings of the clinical aphasiology conference*. Minneapolis: BRK Publishers.

Keenan, J.S., and Brassell, E.G. (1974). A study of factors related to prognosis for individual aphasic patients. *Journal of Speech and Hearing Disorders, 39,* 257–269.

Kertesz, A. (1979). *Aphasia and associated disorders*. New York: Grune and Stratton.

Kertesz, A. (1982). *The western aphasia battery*. New York: Grune and Stratton.

Kertesz, A. (1984a). Recovery from aphasia. In F.C. Rose (Ed.), *Advances in neurology: Progress in aphasiology*. New York: Raven Press.

Kertesz, A. (1984b). Praxis in aphasia. In F.C. Rose (Ed.), *Advances in neurology: Progress in aphasiology*. New York: Raven Press.

Kinsbourne, M. (1971). The minor cerebral hemisphere as a source of aphasic speech. *Archives of Neurology, 25,* 302–306.

Kirby, J. (1978). Blissymbolics and an aphasic patient. *Alberta Speech and Hearing Association Journal, 3,* 4.

Kushner, D., and Winitz, H. (1977). Extended comprehension practice applied to an aphasic patient. *Journal of Speech and Hearing Disorders, 42,* 296–306.

Lane, V.W., and Samples, J.M. (1981). Facilitating communication skills in adult apraxics: Application of Blissymbolics in a group setting. *Journal of Communication Disorders, 14,* 157–167.

LaPointe, L.L. (1977). Base-10 programmed-stimulation: Task specification scoring and plotting performance in aphasia therapy. *Journal of Speech and Hearing Disorders, 42,* 90–105.

LaPointe, L. (1984). Approaches to aphasia treatment. In F. C. Rose (Ed.), *Advances in neurology: Progress in aphasiology.* New York: Raven Press.

LaPointe, L.L., and Horner, J. (1979). *Reading comprehension battery of aphasia.* Tigard, OR: CC Publications.

LeBrun, Y., and Hoops, R. (1974). *Intelligence and aphasia.* Amsterdam: Swets and Zeitlinger.

Lenneberg, E.H. (1967). *Biological foundations of language.* New York: John Wiley and Sons.

Lubinski, R. (1981). Environmental language intervention. In R. Chapey (Ed.), *Language intervention strategies in adult aphasia.* Baltimore: Williams and Wilkins.

McAleese, P.M., Collins, M., Rosenbek, J., and Hengst, J.A. (1984). *Aphasia rehabilitation: Is the result of our efforts a carrot?* Paper presented at the American Speech-Language-Hearing Association National Convention, San Francisco.

McNeil, M.R. (1982). The nature of aphasia in adults. In Lass, J.J., McReynolds, L.V., Northern, J.L., and Yoder, D.E. (Eds.), *Speech, language and hearing, Vol. II: Speech and language pathology.* Philadelphia: W.B. Saunders.

McNeil, M.R., and Prescott, T.E. (1978). *The Revised Token Test.* Baltimore: University Park Press.

McReynolds, L.V., and Kearns, K.P. (1983). *Single subject experimental designs in communicative disorders.* Baltimore: University Park Press.

Malone, M.A. (1978). *Competence communicative behaviors of emergent leaders in small group systems.* Unpublished master's thesis, University of Maine.

Marie, P. (1906). Revision de la question de l'aphasie: L'aphasie de 1861 a 1866: essaie de critique historique sur la genere de la doctrine de Broca. *Semaine Medicale de Paris, 26,* 565–571.

Marquardt, T., Tonkovich, M., and DeVault, S. (1976). Group therapy and stroke club programs for aphasic adults. *Tennessee Speech and Hearing Association Journal, 26,* 2–20.

Marshall, R.C., and King, P.S. (1972). *Effects of fatigue produced by isokinetic exercise upon the communication ability of aphasic patients.* Paper presented at the Conference on Clinical Aphasiology, Albuquerque.

Marshall, R.S. (1979). *Clinician controlled auditory stimulation for aphasic adults.* Tigard, OR: CC Publications.

Marshall, R.S., Tomkins, C.A., Rau, M.T., Phillips, D.S., and Golper, L.A., (1979). Speech and language services for severely aphasic patients: Some professional considerations. In R. Brookshire (Ed.), *Proceedings of the clinical aphasiology conference.* Minneapolis: BRK Publishers.

Mayo Clinic Procedures for Language Evaluation, unpublished.

Meyer, J.S., Kanda, T., Fukuuch, T., Shimazu, K., Dennis, E.W., and Ereiesson, A.D. (1971). Clinical prognosis correlated with hemispheric blood flow in cerebral infarction. *Stroke, 2,* 383–394.

Mills, R. (1982). *Microcomputerized auditory comprehension training.* Paper presented at the Clinical Aphasiology Conference, Oshkosh, WI.

Mohr, J.P., Pessin, M.S., Finkelstein, S., Funkenstein, H.H., Duncan, G.W., and Davis, K.R. (1978). Broca aphasia: Pathologic and clinical. *Neurology, 28,* 311–324.

Moscovitch, M. (1981). Right hemisphere language. *Topics in Language Disorders, 1,* 41–61.

Moss, C.S. (1972). *Recovery with Aphasia*. Urbana, IL: University of Illinois Press.

Mount Sinai Hospital of Cleveland. Picture communication board. Cleo Living Aids, Cleveland, Ohio.

Muma, J.R., and McNeil, M.R. (1981). Intervention in Aphasia: Psychosociolinguistic Perspectives. In R. Chapey (Ed.), *Language intervention strategies in aphasia*. Baltimore: Williams and Wilkins.

National Institutes of Health, Public Health Service (1969). *Human communication and its disorders—an overview.* Washington, DC: National Advisory Neurological Diseases and Stroke Council.

Odell, K., Collins, M., Dirkx, T., and Kelso, D. (1985). *A computerized version of the Coloured Progressive Matrices.* Paper presented the Conference on Clinical Aphasiology, Ashton, OR.

Ojeman, G.A. (1978). Language localization and variability. *Brain and Language, 6,* 239-260.

Ojeman, G.A. (1979). Individual variability in cortical localization of language. *Journal of Neurosurgery, 50,* 164-169.

Paivio, A., and Begg, I. (1981). *Psychology of language.* Englewood Cliffs, NJ: Prentice-Hall.

Pieniadz, J.M., Naeser, M.A., Koff, E., and Levine, H.L. (1983). CT scan cerebral hemispheric asymmetry measurements in stroke cases with global aphasia: Atypical asymmetries associated with improved recovery. *Cortex, 19,* 371-391.

Poeck, K., de Bleser, R., and Graf von Keyserlingk, D. (1984a). Neurolinguistic status and localization of lesion on aphasic patients with exclusively consonant-vowel recurring utterances. *Brain, 107,* 199-218.

Poeck, K., de Bleser, R., and Graf von Keyserlingk, D. (1984b). Computed tomography localization of standard aphasic syndromes. In F.C. Rose (Ed.), *Advances in neurology: Progress in aphasiology.* New York: Raven Press.

Porch, B.E. (1967, 1983). *Porch index of communicative ability.* Palo Alto, CA: Consulting Psychologists Press.

Porch, B.E. (1981). Therapy subsequent to the PICA. In R. Chapey (Ed.), *Language intervention strategies in aphasia.* Baltimore: Williams and Wilkins.

Porch, B.E., and Collins, M.J. (1973). Unpublished data.

Porch, B.E., and Collins, M.J. (1984). *Rating of patients' independence.* Unpublished.

Porch, B.E., Collins, M., Wertz, R.T., and Friden, T. (1980). Statistical prediction of change in aphasia. *Journal of Speech and Hearing Research, 23,* 312-321.

Premack, D. (1971). Language in chimpanzee. *Science, 172,* 808-822.

Raven, J.C. (1962). *Coloured progressive matrices.* London: H.K. Lewis. NY: The Psychological Corporation.

Riese, W. (1970). Cerebral dominance: Its origin, its history, and its nature. *Clio Medica, 5,* 319-326.

Rosenbek, J.C., Collins, M.J., and Wertz, R.T. (1976). Intersystemic reorganization for aphaxia of speech. In R. Brookshire (Ed.), *Proceedings of the conference on clinical aphasiology.* Minneapolis: BRK Publishers.

Rosenbek, J.C., Lemme, M.L., Ahern, M.B., Harris, E.H., and Wertz, R.T. (1973). A treatment for apraxia of speech in adults. *Journal of Speech and Hearing Disorders 38,* 462-472.

Rosenberg, B., and Edwards, A. (1965). An automated multiple response alternative training program for use with aphasics. *Journal of Speech and Hearing Research, 8,* 415–419.

Ross, E.D., and Rush, J. (1981). Diagnosis and neuroanatomical correlates of depression in brain-damaged patients. Implications for a neurology of depression. *Archives of General Psychiatry, 38,* 1344–1354.

Rubens, A. (1977). The role of changes within the central nervous system during recovery from aphasia. In M. Sullivan and M. Kommers (Eds.), *Rationale for adult aphasia therapy.* Lincoln, Nebraska: University of Nebraska Medical Center.

Sanders, S.B., Hamby, E.I., and Nelson, M. (1984). Critical factors associated with the success or failure of community stroke clubs. In R. Brookshire (Ed.), *Proceedings of the conference on clinical aphasiology.* Minneapolis: BRK Publishers.

Sarno, M.T. (1963). *Understanding aphasia: A guide for family and friends.* New York: The Institute of Rehabilitation Medicine, New York University Medical Center.

Sarno, M.T. (1969). *The functional communication profile.* Rehabilitation Monograph 42, New York University Medical Center.

Sarno, M.T., and Levita, E. (1979). Recovery in treated aphasia during the first year post-stroke. *Stroke, 10,* 663–670.

Sarno, M.T., and Levita, E. (1981). Some observations on the nature of recovery in global aphasia. *Brain and Language, 13,* 1–12.

Saya, J.M. (1978). Bliss and the adult aphasic. *Alberta Speech and Hearing Association, 3,* 8.

Schuell, H. (1965). *Minnesota test for differential diagnosis of aphasia.* Minneapolis: University of Minnesota Press.

Schuell, H., Jenkins, J.H., and Jimenez-Pabon, E. (1964). *Aphasia in adults.* New York: Harper and Row.

Searleman, A. (1977). A review of right hemisphere linguistic capabilities. *Psychological Bulletin, 84,* 503–528.

Selnes, O.A. (1976). A note on On representation of language in the right hemisphere of righthanded people. *Brain and Language, 3,* 583–589.

Selnes, O.A., Niccum, N.E., and Rubens, A.B. (1982). CT scan correlates of recovery of auditory comprehension. In R. Brookshire (Ed.), *Proceedings of the conference on clinical aphasiology.* Minneapolis: BRK Publishers.

Skelly, M., Schinsky, L., Smith, R., and Fust, R.S. (1974). American Indian Sign (Amerind) as a facilitator of verbalization for the oral verbal apraxic. *Journal of Speech and Hearing Disorders, 39,* 445–456.

Smith, A. (1972). *Diagnosis, intelligence, and rehabilitation of chronic aphasics: Final report.* Ann Arbor, MI: University of Michigan Department of Physical Medicine and Rehabilitation.

Sparks, R.W. (1981). Melodic Intonation Training. In R. Chapey (Ed.), *Language intervention strategies in aphasia.* Baltimore: Williams and Wilkins.

Sperry, R.W. (1968). Hemispheric deconnection and unity in conscious awareness. *American Psychologist, 23,* 723.

Sperry, R. (1984). Consciousness, personal identity and the divided brain. *Neuropsychologia, 22,* 661–673.

Spinnler, H., and Vignolo, L. (1966). Impaired recognition of meaningful sounds in aphasia. *Cortex, 2,* 337–348.

Stein, S.C. (1981). Medical management of cerebrovascular accidents. In R. Chapey (Ed.), *Language intervention strategies in adult aphasia.* Baltimore:

Williams and Wilkins.

Towey, M.P., and Pettit, J.M. (1980). Improving communicative competence in global aphasia. In R. Brookshire (Ed.), *Proceedings of the conference on clinical aphasiology*. Minneapolis: BRK Publishers.

Van Horn, G., and Hawes, A. (1982). Global aphasia without hemiparesis: A sign of embolic encephalopathy. *Neurology, 32,* 403–406.

Wallace, G.L., and Canter, G.J. (1985). Effects of personally relevant language materials on the performance of severely aphasic individuals. *Journal of Speech and Hearing Disorders, 50,* 385–390.

Wapner, W., and Gardner, H. (1979). A note on patterns of comprehension and recovery in global aphasia. *Journal of Speech and Hearing Research, 22,* 765–772.

Warren, R.L. (1976). Terminating treatment: A round table discussion. In R. Brookshire (Ed.), *Proceedings of the conference on clinical aphasiology*. Minneapolis: BRK Publishers.

Weigl, E., and Bierwisch, M. (1970). Neuropsychology and linguistics: Topics of common research. *Foundations of Language, 6,* 1–18.

Wepman, J.M. (1972). Aphasia therapy: A new look. *Journal of Speech and Hearing Disorders, 2* (37), 203–214.

Wertz, R.T., Collins, M., Weiss, D., Kurtzke, J.F., Friden, T., Brookshire, R.H., Pierce, J., Holtzapple, P., Hubbard, D., Porch, B., West, J., Davis, L., Matovitch, V., Morley, G., Resurrecion, E. (1981). Veterans Administration Cooperative Study on Aphasia: A comparison of individual and group treatment. *Journal of Speech and Hearing Research, 24,* 580–594.

Wilcox, M.J.,and Davis, G. (1977). Speech act analysis of aphasic communication in individual and group settings. In R. Brookshire (Ed.), *Proceedings of the conference on clinical aphasiology*. Minneapolis: BRK Publishers.

Winitz, H., Reeds, J., and Garcia, P. (1975). *Natural language learning* (Vol. 1). Kansas City: General Linguistics.

Zangwill, O.L. (1960). Le probleme de l'apraxie ideatoire. *Revue Neurologique, 102,* 595–603.

# AUTHOR INDEX

# SUBJECT INDEX